MENO MATTERS

How to Master the Menopause

Survive, Thrive and Feel Alive

SHELLEY CHAPMAN

First published in 2018

ISBN: 978-1-9999399-0-8

CONTENTS

TESTIMONIALS

"Shelley has created a powerful hug of a book! It's totally approachable and covers pretty much every aspect of perimenopause and menopause that you can think of, and probably a few you haven't! It dives straight into the lived experience of being a *person* while experiencing menopause and has the inspiring message that menopause can be the start of a new beginning, a coming into our true selves. Not something to just get through but something that launches us as the powerful, fearless creatures we all are inside! It's structured so you can dip in and dip out as you need and has a clear place in your 'living life the way you want to' arsenal. Thank you Shelley!"

Gayle Johnson, gayle@redtreewriting.com

"This book is a little gem and just the antidote to all the negative menopause chatter... it really makes you want to live for NOW even with menopause symptoms!"

Laura Brennan

"Not having my Mum around to discuss the menopause, I enjoyed this cheery view on the menopause, it was like a chat with my Mum"

Nancy Detchon

"What a gem - this little book is very informative on all matters concerning the menopause. The writer draws from her own experience, that of friends and plenty of research to bring a concise easy read that is packed full of useful tips on managing the menopause."

Julie Jepsom

"Shelley has written a very honest account of dealing with the menopause before, during and after. Speaking from her own experiences, she's dealt with every aspect menopausal women go through. Her wonderful humour has also added a light hearted element to the book making you feel it's OK and you're not on your own. You can refer back to it time after time - a definite bedside read! Shelley you are an inspiration! – I loved it"

Margaret Brobbin

"I found this so useful to pick up and read a chapter or section because it gave practical advice in a friendly and amusing manner. I can't wait for the next quirky look at life! I love it."

Christine Eley

"Shelley has given women, whether they are on, yet to be on or have reached the end of their menopause journey an invaluable insight into all kinds of advice and tips to enhance an often low and difficult time in their lives.

Speaking as someone who has reached the end of my menopause journey, I was amazed at how much was still pertinent to me. Thank you Shelley"

Jan Jones

"This book is a 'must-read' for any man who, like me, has no previous understanding of menopause and how it affects your partner or relatives. Once you have read the book you will have a far greater understanding of how your actions can make things much smoother and a lot calmer for those who are going through the menopause. It's a highly recommended read!"

Richard Anthony

DISCLAIMER

The information contained in this book is general in nature and for informational purposes. It is not meant to substitute the advice provided by your own Doctor or other Medical Professional.

None of the statements in this book are a recommendation as to how to treat any particular disease or health-related condition. If you suspect you have a disease or health-related condition of any kind, you should contact your Doctor immediately.

Please read all product packaging carefully and it is advised that you consult with a Healthcare Professional before starting any diet, exercise, supplementation or medication program.

Cosmetic products have not been evaluated by the Food and Drug Administration and are not intended to diagnose, treat, cure, or prevent disease.

DEDICATION

This book is dedicated to *you*, because you've picked it up, read or browsed a bit of it and decided it can help you in some way, or a lot of ways, through this menopausal journey that you've no choice but to be on.

This is *your personal journal*, because we're all different and unique in our own way, especially with the menopause and this is *your* journey and for you to find what works for you…

It's so you can pass this down to your daughters or granddaughters and make their menopausal journey a lot easier.

Your book is peppered with all sorts of tips and advice and it's my mission to help you with as much as I can and in as many areas as you need, so that we can see what works for you, so that you get the life you truly desire and deserve.

I've come through the menopausal journey and am nearly out the other side. Learnt so much that really helped and made it easy, but took me longer to find out, so that's why you now hold this journal.

There are pages and areas where you will want to write things down, that are personal to you… Why have I done this?

Because it's an insight and an important piece of you, to pass down to them, at a time when they will really need it. Because what's worked for you, should work for them too.

It would have made all the difference to me with my journey, if I had known what to expect and what my mother, or even grandmother had gone through and I wouldn't have felt so alone.

This is YOUR book, YOUR journey, and YOUR story.

Your name ……………………………………………………………………

My message to you my darling …

ACKNOWLEDGMENTS

Thank you Russ, my amazing husband and best friend, for being with me for 43 years and especially during my Menopausal journey. Thank you for your love, strength, patience, and above all, support whilst I found the "New Me". I love you with my all heart and soul, you're not only my rock, but the wind beneath my wings.

To Andrew Reynolds for being the start of this incredible journey that I'm now on, and bringing the sort of people into my world that I didn't even know existed.

To Helena Holrick, thank you for being the person that showed me the direction I should go in, which then made the difference to the path I followed.

To Steven and Corrina Essa, who opened up the World to me expanding 'the dream' into reality and showed me how to put it together through the amazing...

Grace Heart, who helped me so much in realising the dream. Thank you for your support, encouragement and unwavering belief in me, this book, and The Menopause Help Programme that you helped me put together, to be able to reach women worldwide. What an incredible ride it's been.

Laura Brennan for all your support, being so easy to talk to and above all for the fantastic illustrations for this book. May there be many more x

And to the lovely Kevin Bunting for putting me in sight of that amazing inspirational tree at Theobalds Park that allowed me so easily to put this book together.

To Simon Coulson (Internet Business School) where I was introduced to Rick McMunn – (link on page 176) who literally brought me to print and on Amazon. What an amazingly quick ride it's been, but so enjoyable and you do exactly what you promise – incredible!

PREFACE

This little book, now *your* little book, is full of snippets of information, bite sized for you to digest and think about. This is not a lecture or a YOU MUST DO book, but something that covers topics and subjects that affect us ladies with things that you might not know, or might want to try.

Not only that, it's also a journal, so that you can write down what matters to you or has helped you and then see how it can help you with becoming the woman you want to be, the 'New You'.

The chapters are in no particular order, so you can either read it, cover to cover, or just flick through it, because there's something on every page that will help you and I'm hoping that no matter where you open the page and stick the pin in, you'll learn something.

But firstly, I must warn you that this book isn't going to moan about the Menopause because that doesn't help you, or your symptoms.

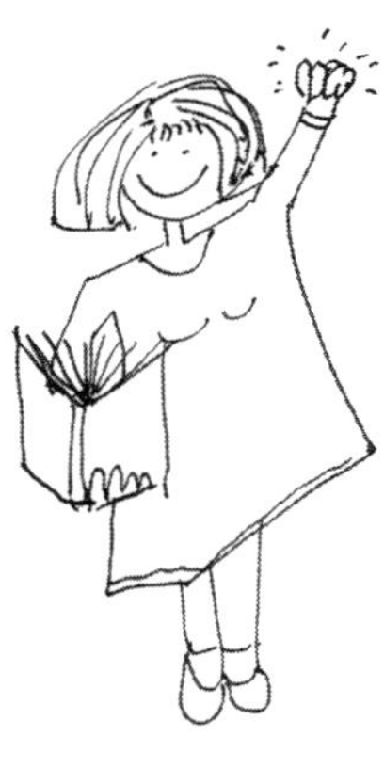

It's about some things that can really help you through not only this stage of your life, but how you can also enjoy the many chapters of your life that are to come.

You might be wondering what gives me the authority to write this book and talk to you about the menopause – well I've been menopausal now for 15 years after an emergency hysterectomy and decided it wasn't going to change my life in any way, in fact I was going to use this time to grow and become the sort of woman that I wanted to be from now on in, but more of that in chapter 26.

This little book covers some of the things that either I do, or I've found out about that help other women, so it's quite diverse because we're all different and no two women go through the menopause in the same way. I've found out loads more, so hopefully that's for the next book that I'll write.

I'll be talking to you about how you can manage (naturally) a lot of your symptoms.

I'll also talk to you about how you can manage yourself, your body, your thoughts, emotions and to take back control of YOU.

How can I make such dramatic a statement? *Because I've done it for me* and countless other women and our lives are so much more different, better and happier and I honestly want the same for you too.

But this one was written for *you*, so welcome my lovely friend and follow me on a journey that I hope will change a lot of things for you, in a good way.

1
This is for You

So let's get you off on the right foot, straight away and make this your personal book and journey

In some of the chapters, you will need to write things down so that you can focus on what you want and how you would like your life to change in that area.

Let me start by saying… you are amazing! – not in a weird way, but in what you do every day, every week of just about every year!

Like most women, you most probably juggle work, home and family doing everything in your power to make your family's life run as smoothly as possible. Just take a moment to look back at what you've achieved (I'll bet you've never had a moment to *really* realise just how much you *have* achieved!).

So, to get you in the right mind set, right from the start, please have a think and write here, 3 of your best achievements.

1) ....

....

2) ....

....

3) ....

....

Right, holding that thought, I want you to know that there's very little that can stop you with how you want your future to be.

It just needs an idea or two as to which step or direction you want to take first and mould it around your circumstances in the present moment and then change it as your life changes and more time or opportunities come along. This really is a dip in, dip out book, depending on what you want, when you want it.

I've been asked so many times "does the Menopause matter? Honestly, is anyone really interested in what I'm going through?" Of course it does. It's real and encroaches into just about every aspect of your everyday life.

Some of us suffer more with it, some less. But I want you to realise, RIGHT NOW, that it's not the beginning of the end, but the beginning of *one of the best chapters of your life!* It's the beginning of the rest of your life, literally, and that's why this journal of yours is so important, this is *your* journey to a "New You".

Did you know that women's attitude to ageing has changed from our mother's time? The rule book has sort of been thrown away and that's a good thing. Things like 'Empty Nest' and 'Menopause' 'That Time of Life', used to send women into a downward spiral that their most useful years were over. BUT NOT NOW…

A lot of women are now looking at this time as the perfect excuse to *reinvent* themselves – a la Madonna! Ok, I'm not saying you have to go to that extreme, but when you start seeing some of the women on our screens who are menopausal and refuse to let it dull their life, but embrace it and start making differences to the way they look and feel, you'll see just how powerful this little journal of yours is going to be.

They now do things they always wanted to do but didn't think they had the time, or had convinced themselves that they were too old to start.

To go shopping and choose things that they love, rather than what's practical.

That it's actually ok to be a bit selfish and think of themselves first for a change and you know what? A lot of us are really, *really* enjoying the difference this change of thinking is making.

Some do it with a bang, some with baby steps, but it doesn't matter. As long as the journey is *your* journey and makes *you* happy.

This next chapter of your life is a long one, but it's yours, so let's make it a happy rather than a lonely one. You're never too old to make a start, make a difference or be happy.

I'll mention now (to reinforce just that point) that we spend 50% of our adult life as a postmenopausal female! FIFTY PERCENT!! So that means that you've got far more time, after the menopause, to do so many of the things that you really want to do.

And you know what?

As you get older you can get away with so much more than you could when you were younger! Why? I think it's because we can actually do more 'under the radar' and people's attention isn't on us as much as we think it is, so we can just go for it!

Read on and get some ideas, and a few laughs. We all deserve to have the sort of life we want and it's not as difficult as you think!

Ok, let's get the nasty stuff out of the way and talk about the menopause, and then we can move onto all the other things that you can do that'll make your life just get better and better…

NOTES: Use this space to write down the areas of your life that you'd like to make changes in…

2
Are You Menopausal or Going Nuts?

The Menopause in a Nutshell...

Look at it as puberty in reverse! Mother Nature is trying to get rid of all the things that you no longer need, to cleanse you from the inside if you like, so that you no longer have to worry about getting periods and getting pregnant. It takes a while for you to get to your 50's (age 51 is the usual time for women to start the menopause, although some start earlier – either naturally or by having a full hysterectomy, and some a bit later).

Just about every woman will experience the menopause, but each of us is unique in how we'll experience it. Some will get mild symptoms, some moderate and some more severe.

Remember, THERE ARE NO RULES, but how you deal with it both mentally (your attitude) and with the treatment choices that you use (which will include a huge variety of alternative remedies and lifestyle adjustments), will determine how easy or more difficult it is for you to cope with *your* menopause journey.

So be patient with Mother Nature as it's going to take a while for her to sort everything out, but, honestly, it's worth the wait!

So what exactly is the menopause?

It's when the decreasing levels of the hormone that we have, called Estrogen, causes your ovaries to stop producing eggs and this causes the most typical symptoms of the menopause like...

Hot Flushes (or Chills),

Night Sweats

Mood Swings

Aches and Pains in your joints as your suppleness decreases.

Some women might experience flavours differently, like a Metallic, or Vinegary taste in their mouth and this is an indication that the menopause is on its way.

Your Periods will be all over the place as well. Your normal cycle that you're used to will become irregular and also you might experience heavy bleeding. It's not until 12 months + have passed without you having a period that you're considered in the menopause, but it has been known for some women to get to nearly 16 months, and yep, another period comes along. So in a nutshell, your periods get really weird until they finally stop and remember, it's still possible to fall pregnant during this time!!

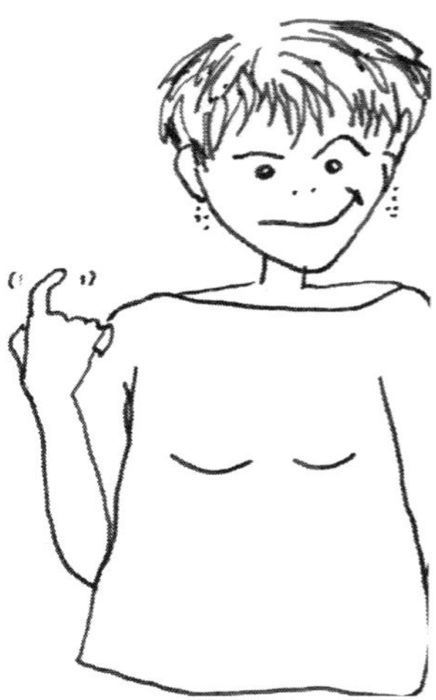

As hard as it is, just try and be patient and concentrate on other areas of your life, rather than your symptoms (but I'll cover more about this a bit later). Why do I say this? Because the more you concentrate on your symptoms, the more acute they seem to become and the more this could pull you down. In psychological terms it's called 'selective attention', so if you look for red cars, you suddenly see loads of red cars!

Let me explain…

Remember when you felt unwell, but you had to go out, or go to work? You coped with the day, became distracted, in fact, you got to the end of the day and noticed that you'd hardly even thought about it, until you got home and had the time to consider how you were feeling and – guess what – all your symptoms came back with a vengeance!

There are other things that can happen and I'll go through some of those now, to get them out of the way…

You could experience Anxiety, Itchy Skin, Eyes, Mouth and/or Vaginal Dryness. Your skin starts to dry and the elasticity in it drops so you'll notice Wrinkles start to appear (oh marvellous), but it's not irreparable and more of that later.

Just be aware that some menopause symptoms can last an average of 7 years, but some women can have them for as long as 14 or so!

STOP!!!

I'm not telling you anymore at this point, because this is a POSITIVE book about the menopause, not a NEGATIVE one, and those symptoms that I've listed above have remedies that can deal with them – even wrinkles! So it's best that you forget about or learn how to deal with your symptoms, so that you can enjoy LIFE. This is the only one you have so just go for it.

You can do this!

So you need to look at the menopause and after it – "After Life" in a different way than you have with everyday life. Why? Because this book is dealing with you and only you. You have to concentrate now on yourself for once and realise your body is changing and to do everything you can to look forward to your life from now on in.

This will all be for the better, I promise you, but before you get to that 'Light at the End of the Tunnel' moment, it's my job, in this book, to prepare you as best I can to deal with some of your symptoms, but more importantly, how you deal and cope with the Menopause and come out of it a very different and most wonderful version of you.

Because when you realise that you're not alone, (at the time of writing there's 13 million menopausal women in the UK alone!), that just about every female on our planet is going through, will, or has, gone through the menopause and come out the other side.

It's not as scary as you think it will be and there is so much to look forward to. That's because the best way to look at this phase of your life is as becoming the 'New You', totally liberated and with so much to look forward to. The Japanese look at it as their 'second spring' and that's what this time should be for you too, a second chance to live and have the life that you want.

I need you to concentrate on the fact that you don't become less of a woman – you actually become more of one (now don't pull that face!). A woman who is eventually free and liberated from those pesky hormones, period cramps, etc... and more empowered.

Don't believe me? Well it's happened to me and countless other women and if you want to join us – WE'RE HAVING THE TIME OF OUR LIVES...

← I CAN / I CAN'T →

Guess what? Either way you're right!

Did you know that 55% of women aged 45-65 are more confident that they were a decade ago?

Why?

How?

Because they took a deep breath and 'went for it' and found that life actually got more exciting and their lives got better. Life is way too short to live with regret, so honestly, what have you got to lose?

Oh. You might want to know at this point that there's a chapter or two where I cover MEN! Not MENopause, but our partners, husbands, MEN.

It's so that you can show all of this book, or just those relevant chapters to him, if you think it'll help him understand what you're going through. I'll leave it up to you...

See? It's as simple as that – you taking control of what you want to do in this moment, so you can start focusing on yourself and how you're going to deal with this stage of your life...

Write 5 things you (or your partner) won't miss (with you having no period pains/monthly and hormonal changes).

1) ....

2) ....

3) ....

4) ....

5) ....

3
Your Favourite Position
(don't worry, I mean sleep!)

This is a less chatty chapter but has some "hands on'', tried and tested, practical help for you to consider or try...

Now come on, admit it! We all love a good night's sleep and when you're warm and relaxed in a comfy bed, now is the time that you need to tell yourself about the importance of sleep.

Why? Because a good night's sleep can help you stay slim – seriously!

How? Having too little sleep hampers your metabolism and because of this, it contributes to weight gain and quality sleep is an important contributor to weight loss.

So try and get into a routine of going to bed earlier so that you are asleep for longer. You'll know when you've got this cracked, because you'll wake up naturally rather than from an alarm. It might take a while, but persevere, because that, on top of a healthy eating and active lifestyle, will have a very positive effect on you losing weight.

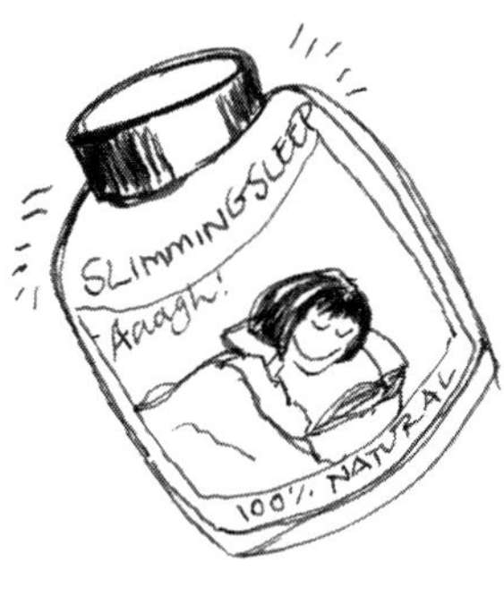

Leave your phone and/or iPad in another room, even better, in the kitchen where it's too far away to be tempted to see it, because it'll still be there in the morning, waiting for you when the kettle's boiling for your morning cuppa!

Not only that, the 'blue' light they emit stimulates your brain waves and you then can't relax and go to sleep, because your brain has now totally woken up and prevents you reaching deep sleep by 3 hours. So if you've been looking at a screen up to 10pm, you won't get quality sleep until 1 am!

Or if you must have your phone or tablet with you in the bedroom, then set it to night time setting after 6pm.

But you could try this! Instead of your phone or tablet, get a good book, lie back, relax and read... it really works! I've read the same chapter 5 times because I've fallen asleep so quickly! It might take a few times to retrain your body, but it won't need much encouragement.

Also, when you go to bed, don't have your room too warm as you'll spend a lot of the night sticking your leg out from under the duvet, trying to cool down & disrupting your 'stay slim' sleep pattern!

Make your room cool by leaving your radiators off or on very low, maybe just keep the bathroom towel rail on and open the window just before you go to bed, as long as there are no midges around!

Make *you* cool, by wearing as little as possible, because when a night sweat comes on, your clothing will just stick to you. But if you throw the covers off, then it's just your skin that has to cool down. If you do sweat a lot, then maybe put a large towel under your bottom sheet which you can change easily.

As I said before, if you can go to bed at the same time each night, this will get you and your body into a routine.

Make sure you have comfy pillows and bedding that's easy to kick off and then pull back on if you happen to have a night sweat.

Putting a pillow under your knees is also a good thing to try, it takes the pressure off your back and because it gives you the feeling of comfort and softness, it helps with something to relax into and it's easier to fall asleep.

Cut down on your alcohol before bed because women have less water in their bodies than men, so when we have some alcohol, more of it goes directly into our blood stream (compared to a man, where it ends up in body water), which is why it has a disruptive effect on our sleep patterns.

So drink any alcohol in moderate amounts and long enough before bed for your last glass, because even though you think it'll make you feel tired and relax you, it actually stimulates your brain and makes it harder to have the right sort of sleep.

Which means, when you do go to bed and fall asleep, you might find that you wake up a couple or so hours later, then not being able to switch off because your brain has started to wake up, so you lay there, tossing and turning and trying not to think of all the things you need to do tomorrow.

Another thing that you need to avoid to have a good night's sleep is coffee. It takes at least 8 hours for your last cup of coffee to be out of your system and is a huge stimulant for your brain. So if you go to bed at 10pm, your last coffee should be at 2pm so that it's not still in your system.

So having something like a hot chocolate instead will relax you and your brain so that everything is prepared for your bedtime routine and SLEEP.

As we age we lose Magnesium and this really is important for your body, in lots of ways. It's a mineral our body needs and affects different areas, and for lots of women, interrupted sleep is quite a problem during the menopause.

Why do I mention Magnesium in this chapter (well I mention it a lot actually), it's because some women, when they take Magnesium Citrate, (max 350mg/day) 1 hour before going to bed, or have a warm bath with Magnesium flakes in (Epsom Salts), it really helps them sleep.

It's important though that you MUST consult your Doctor before taking Magnesium if you're on any medication as this could interfere with what you've been prescribed, or if you have kidney issues, thyroid or high blood pressure etc.

Another thing you could try, if you're still finding it difficult dropping off to sleep because you've got so much on your mind, is do a brain dump!

Whilst you're drinking your hot chocolate, write a list of all the things you want to do tomorrow, highlight the top three that have to be done and then it's out of your head and you don't need to worry about it as the list will be ready for you when you come down for your morning cuppa.

But if you're worried that you'll think of something as soon as you go to bed, then have a pad and pencil on the bedside table, quickly write it down if it comes to mind (without switching the light on if you can manage) and then lie back, relax and sleep.

What has worked for a lot of women, when they wake up with night sweats and then their brain thinks it's time to get up, is this... the 4:7:8 method

Take a deep breath in for 4 counts

Hold for 7 counts

Breath out over 8 counts and relax into your comfy bed as you do so.

Doing this prevents your brain from kicking in as it's so busy focusing on counting and relaxing and will soon get the message and sleep will envelop you.

Get into the habit of drinking a pint of water before you go to bed (it won't take long for your bladder to get used to it) because your body does it's mending whilst you're asleep and this is exactly what it needs to help plump your skin out. So don't be surprised if you wake up with your skin looking younger than when you went to bed!

NOTES: Write here what you've tried and what has worked for you…

4
Let's Iron Out Your Wrinkles!

You know us women moan about our 'laughter lines' as being wrinkles or crows' feet? Well how about totally turning that way of looking at them on its head and rather see them as being 'happiness lines', (because it took a lot of smiling and laughing to get them there) and smile each time you look at your reflection. You'll see just how beautiful you really are!

But there are some things you can do about minimising them, and those I'll cover in a minute.

There's nothing more attractive than a woman with a happy smile. It makes you look younger, fun and carefree – why would you not want to look younger each day? People are drawn to happy people… it has a knock-on effect.

BUT THERE'S MORE…

Unfortunately, our eyes show our age because they're the first to show signs of ageing, due to the fact that the area under our eyes can have a biological age of up to 22 years older than the rest of our face!

This is because the skin is weaker and less elastic than the skin on our face, which is why you have to be so gentle when applying cream around your eye area, so 'pat' it on gently with your ring finger, rather than spread it on (which can stretch the skin).

Find a cream that's specifically for eyes as these will be different than the creams for the rest of your face. Do they really make a difference? Yes, they do, because these are produced for the skin around our eyes.

They're thicker and usually have more oil than regular facial creams have, as the skin, especially under your eyes, stops producing oil and therefore dries out a lot more quickly If you use it every day, you'll start to see a difference and people will start to notice too!

So, maybe do as I do and carry in your handbag, a hydrating eye cream and during the day re-apply it by patting it, especially under your eyes and up the side, again using your ring finger so you don't stretch the delicate skin.

You screw your eyes up a lot during the day, and especially if it's windy or cold, or sometimes by just rubbing them, so by re-applying it during the day your eyes will appear to have fewer wrinkles and this will go a long way to reducing any more in the future.

Do you want to know what works like MAGIC at night and got rid of the wrinkles around my eyes (well, until I smile or laugh)? Coconut Oil... The 100% Pure Coconut Oil that you can cook with!! You have no idea how amazing this jar of magic is.

After cleansing, use it lightly as a night time moisturiser on your face, neck and chest. It works wonders on all these areas, making the wrinkles on your face a lot lighter (some of them disappear altogether). Your neck will become less wrinkled and dry and it really helps to reduce that 'old handbag' look that some women can get on their chest. Incredible!! It'll be our secret (wink).

Talking about night time – did you know that you can minimize your face and neck wrinkles whilst you sleep? How? By keeping your neck stretched upwards, sleeping on a high-density contour foam pillow that moulds to your shape and gives you maximum support.

This, I'm told, works because it helps prevent wrinkles from forming on your face and neck whilst you're asleep. This is because of the angle that your head is on the pillow – gently stretched more upward than scrunched downward - which can happen using a normal pillow without support!

Something that will really help and will also go a long way to reducing any bags under your eyes is water, and lots of it! Our body is made up of about 70% water and this is vital to keep everything healthy and in order, especially our skin.

So drink a minimum of 2 litres (3 is better) a day and just see the difference in your skin! If this absolutely horrifies you with the amount, have 2 x 1 litre containers and know that you have to try and get through 2-3 of those a day! Why 2?...

Cold water burns more calories than warm, so keep one in the fridge and have the other one so you see it constantly and are reminded to drink as many sips as you can. As soon as it starts getting warm, swap it with the one in the fridge.

On the chart below, track your water intake (litres per day) and write down when you started to see or feel the results of drinking more water and where. Whichever method suits you, visual or measurement (cm's is a good way, rather than inches).

Week 1	Mon	Tue	Wed	Thu	Fri	Sat	Sun	Results
Week 2	Mon	Tue	Wed	Thu	Fri	Sat	Sun	Results
Week 3	Mon	Tue	Wed	Thu	Fri	Sat	Sun	Results
Week 4	Mon	Tue	Wed	Thu	Fri	Sat	Sun	Results
Week 5	Mon	Tue	Wed	Thu	Fri	Sat	Sun	Results
Week 6	Mon	Tue	Wed	Thu	Fri	Sat	Sun	Results

5
Is a New Hairstyle What You Need?

It's sometimes difficult to accept that we're getting older and as we do, we look back on our younger selves, (especially in photos) and wonder what we would have or could have changed - especially with some of the hair styles that we had that were really "trendy". I look at some of my old photos and absolutely cringe at how flipping awful I looked, I mean, what *was* I thinking?

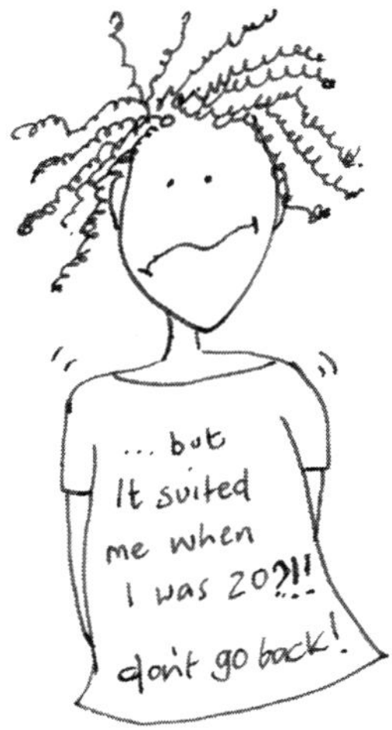
... but
It suited
me when
I was 20?!!
don't go back!

But at the time we would have changed nothing, because that's exactly what we wanted to be – 'trendy'.

But now you have the wisdom of honesty and the knowledge that you can change anything if you really want to and that being a certain age doesn't mean that you have to look a certain way. Absolutely not!

I grant you, sometimes it's easier to just accept your lot, shrug and say "oh well, I'm getting older, so why bother?".

Or you can make yourself a promise that you'll try, one step at a time, to make small changes at first, get your courage back and do something for you, so why not start with your hairstyle?

Are you bored and fed up with your hair?

Have you had the same hairstyle for years and fancy a change?

Whether you want to cut or grow your hair (having spoken to a few hairdressers), this is what the 'pro's' have told me and would love you to do...

Go into some hairdressers local to you and ask them what *they* would do with your hair.

The right stylist for you will take into consideration your lifestyle (the time you can spend on your hair), your hair texture, your face shape etc. Ask them to show you pictures and then decide for yourself what you like, even going away and having a think first if you're still not sure.

It could be so exiting to take control and do something a bit different that maybe you've always privately wanted to do. Either treat yourself or ask for it as a present! The hairdressers are the experts, they want the best for you and you're a walking advert for them, so have fun and do something just for you.

If you're not used to going to the hairdressers it can be a bit daunting picking the right one for you. So another thing you could try, is if you've got a friend whose hair cut or styles you've always loved, ask her where she goes to have hers done.

Or (as I've done on a couple of occasions) when I've fancied a change and passed a woman in the street and thought "wow, I love her style", I've actually gone up and said how much I love it and if she didn't mind, telling me where she has it done? They are normally so taken aback that another woman actually loves how they look, that they willingly tell you, not only the hairdresser, but the name of the stylist also!

So, when you know where to go, make an appointment, ask their advice and see what they think might suit you and just go for it, it's very liberating and a fantastic way to start the journey to the "New You" and for a lot of women, this has been the best way to get the 'ball rolling' as it instantly makes you feel better about yourself.

Unfortunately, one of the symptoms of menopause is thinning or limp hair. Have you got this and it's frustrating you as to how you can get some sort of style that you can manage?

Don't despair, there's loads of things you can do. Try applying a small amount of product like mousse to the roots of towel dried hair, or 'lifting powder' to dry hair. This will give you a much fuller, more glamorous look when you style your hair.

If you use a hairdryer or hot irons to finalise your style, use a heat protecting spray first, one that's designed for high heat (which acts for your hair the same way as immersing your hands in very hot water with rubber gloves on), so that the hot air from the hairdryer or heat from the irons doesn't burn your hair (which can cause it to break). This is a simple solution for a new and maintainable look.

If you're getting grey hair, this can come through coarser and dryer, but don't let that hold you back, because 'coarser' can be really handy when it comes to styling. So fancy a change? How about going shorter and choppier (like a pixie look), it might knock years off you and give you a new zest for life. And if you don't like it – you can always grow it again!

The other thing you could consider, if your hair is coming through grey and you don't like it, is to consider having highlights or lowlights. These, done professionally, can completely transform your hair and its texture.

Are you worried that you're getting a furrowed or lined forehead? Again, menopause causes our skin to dry out and one of the first places we see this is our forehead, because we frown more, it's always open to the elements, or just due to the stress of going through the menopause.

On the subject of forehead wrinkles, a couple of solutions for you would be to use Coconut Oil as a night time moisturiser, as from personal experience with myself and the women I work with, this has a HUGE effect on lessening lines and wrinkles.

In fact, one woman I worked with, used it and in a matter of a few weeks, looked very noticeably younger!

Another thing you could consider is having a hairstyle with a fringe over your brow as (according to the experts) it can be 'extremely de-ageing, can soften a face and hide a bad hairline'. Don't make it heavy though as this can look a bit too severe, so go for something light and feathery.

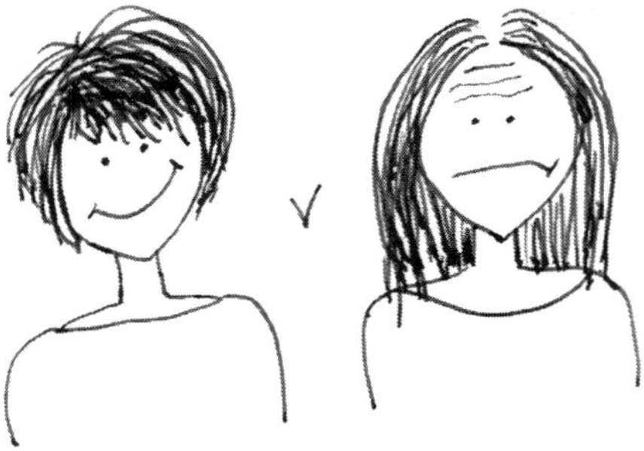

You could part your hair further over, which can really create a soft look, but not to the point of a comb over!

I'm repeating this one (as you'll see below) because it's so important to us ladies and can have such a devastating effect but, as we get menopausal, one of the things that can happen is that your hair thins or falls out. This is because the follicle goes dormant, resting for a while and then starts growing again in a few weeks.

The problem with ageing, is that as we get older, the dormant period gets longer and the growing time gets shorter. So, more hair appears in the plug hole and your scalp gets more visible. The speed of this can be down to genetics, or maybe not, but either way, it's incredibly distressing.

Mine started falling out, you could see my scalp, so I know how distressing it is. I also knew it wasn't genetics as my mother still had a fine head of hair when she died (aged 49) and I could remember her mother having great hair too. I even started wearing a wig but then decided to try a natural remedy to see if that would work and it did...

With incredible results.

In just a few weeks my hair started to grow back and after a few months it was thicker and better than before and still is. The magic pill? Sea Kelp. I take 2 tablets daily and have never looked back. There's a lot of magic to be found in natural remedies, but more of that later.

NOTES: What did you try and what worked for you?

6
You Couldn't Make It Up – Or Could You?

Well, you could actually and you can grow older so elegantly (just like Helen Mirren for example). It's easier than you think. I'm sure she doesn't wake up looking as glamorous as we normally see her, none of us do.

So there's a lot for you to read in this chapter, because there are a lot of makeup products out there that can really help us, especially as we get older.

How about you take yourself off for a treat and go to a department store and ask one of the beauty counters (choose one that's in your price range) to show you how to apply makeup for the look that you're happy with.

Daytime/Evening/Soft/Wow. They will love the fact that you're showing such an interest and will happily tell you anything you want to know.

Or why don't you do it with a friend and enjoy a good day out together. Treat yourself, it's a great confidence booster and be happy – again, do something just for you.

Another thing I've noticed is that as we get older, wearing less makeup on our skin keeps it looking fresh and is less ageing. When I went for a 'beauty makeover' for a special occasion, they put a lot more makeup on than I normally do and I really noticed how it 'sat' in my wrinkles, enhancing them and actually making me look older than I liked. So if you have it done, maybe ask if they could tone it down a bit and make it more natural.

There's loads of choice if you want a bit of colour on your face, or to help hide any blemishes and that's with a soft foundation, tinted moisturiser, BB creams (Beauty Balm, a lighter foundation), CC creams (Complexion Corrector) and DD creams (Daily Defence or Dynamic Do-all).

With any creams that you put on your face, try and get them with an SPF 30 to protect your skin. Try them out on the back of your hand and see which one you prefer. I've always found this useful, especially if it conceals the age spots on my hand, then I know it's going to work for my face!

Correctly applied, it can smooth your complexion which will make it look younger and fresher again, so how do you apply the product correctly? I found this out from the pro's, which was a good thing, as I had been doing it completely the wrong way. The secret to getting a nice soft finish is to use a dampened sponge, or 'stipple' foundation brush and to use a small amount of foundation or tinted moisturiser.

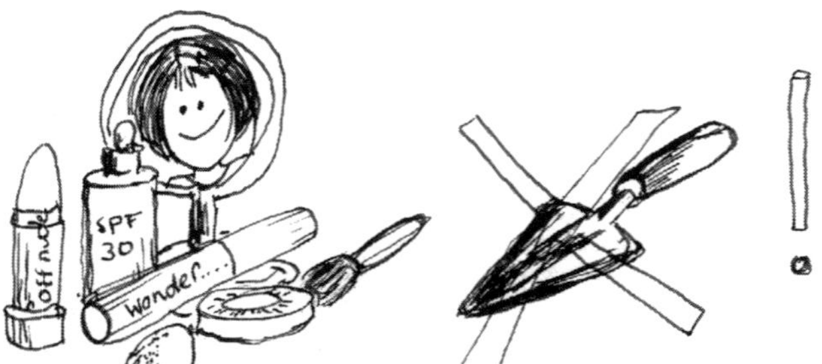

Do you wear foundation but find that as you're getting older and the menopause is changing your skin, it doesn't look as good as it used to? Then try using a Primer first. This will help blur your wrinkles, pores and blemishes. It also gives your foundation or tinted moisturiser a good base to sit on and makes it last longer. Plus, it gives your skin extra protection from the elements - Perfect!

A word of advice though, don't rely on these creams to give your skin the protection it needs throughout the year, especially from the sun. As you get older, your skin will thin more and you need to do as much as you can to prevent it drying out, burning, getting more wrinkles, age spots or, like on your lips, even cancer. So use a sunscreen always, after your moisturiser preferably with an SPF 30 as minimum.

Even though the menopause can cause us to get acne... are you getting spots after using your eyeshadow, blusher brushes, or any makeup brush for that matter? It might be due to the fact that they need a 'bath'. This, I was told, should be at least every month to get rid of skin irritating oil, bacteria and mildew!

Gently 'swish' the brush hair in soapy water (mild shampoo). Immediately rinse thoroughly and squeeze out the water, then rearrange the hairs to their normal shape. Dry naturally with the head of the brushes hanging over the edge of a shelf. They'll be like new and hopefully your skin won't break out in spots, but if hairs on the brush are falling out when you wash it, then it's now too old and you need to replace it.

And on the subject of brushes, as with most things, you get what you pay for. So it's a good idea to spend as much as you can on good brushes (the ones you use the most) as not only will these last a lot longer, your makeup will look a lot better too because of the ability of the brushes to blend better.

If your eyebrows are getting a bit sparse, there's a few things you can do about this like tattooing, micro-dermabrasion or the easiest is to gently comb them into place with any eyebrow comb and use an eyebrow pencil (they range from grey to dark brown) and very softly colour them in, then gently go over them again with the comb to blend the colour so they look as natural as possible. I say softly, because if you do it more firmly they won't look natural, just heavy, and that's not a good look.

Then just use a hint of blusher on your cheeks, define your lashes with mascara and then, of course, a bit of lippy and especially lip balm. You should always use a lip balm, even in the winter - protect, protect, protect because our lips lack the waterproofing outer layer that skin has and are devoid of oil-producing sebaceous glands. This means that they're sensitive to moisture loss, especially in dry, cold air.

Your lips are also susceptible to sunburn since they lack melanin, the pigment that helps shield skin from the sun. Lip cancers are prevalent, Google images of them and you'll know why I mentioned it, it certainly shocked me, because I didn't know that lip cancer existed! It's not nice but so preventable.

So it makes sense to ensure your balm or lipstick contains an SPF too, particularly when in the mountains, in fact, get into the habit of using it all the time. Carry it around in your handbag so you never forget.

If you're confused about what colour lipstick you should go for, then for a truly flattering/natural look that always works, choose a colour that is a step stronger than your own natural lip colour. If you're not quite sure what that is, bite your lips (it will enhance their natural colour) and match the lipstick colour to them now.

NOTES: What did you try? What difference did it make? How did it make you feel?

7
How You Can Control Anxiety

Easier said than done right?

But oddly enough, and a lot of women don't know this, Anxiety can be a common problem coming up to and during the menopause. Some women can get it mildly, others can suffer from it quite badly and it happened to me.

I started getting anxious, completely out of the blue! Horrible, worrying and I also thought that something was wrong with me. So if this is happening to you too, worry not, because there are a few things that might help, so see which one works for you...

As soon as I found out that Anxiety is one of the more common menopausal symptoms us poor women can suffer with, I found out that what a lot of women do, when they feel anxious, or have a feeling of dread, is tell themselves quite firmly "It's just the menopause" and do you know what? For a lot of women that works and the feeling soon goes away because they know it's the menopause and not them (if that makes sense?). The power of the mind is HUGE.

Or, try going for a walk as exercise relaxes and de-stresses you. Distract yourself – identify to yourself when you don't feel anxious and make that happen more often.

If that doesn't work for you then you could try something else...

If 'talking firmly' to yourself isn't working, then I found something that really worked for me and for other women too who suffer from mild to moderate Anxiety.

It's Magnesium... again... and worked for me, just about instantly!

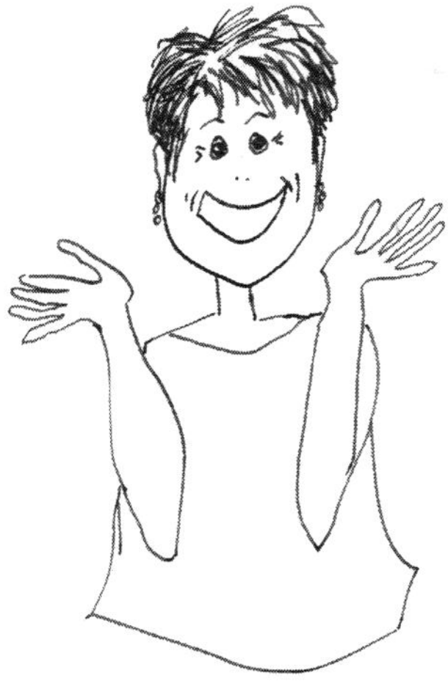

Why Magnesium? Because, in a nutshell (according to ods.od.nih.gov), there have been several pieces of evidence that link low Magnesium to ageing and we become Magnesium deficient.

A 350mg (no higher) supplement of Magnesium Citrate (as it's easily absorbed by your body) every day is worth trying if you suffer from mild to moderate Anxiety, it works for me and all my Anxiety went!

It's also meant to help with sleeping and because your body needs it every day try taking 1 x 150mg in the morning and one at night before bed.

But like I said before, if you're on any medication, you must check with your Doctor first before taking it, just in case it reacts with what you've been prescribed, or if you have any kidney issues, thyroid or high blood pressure etc.. Plus, a Doctor is the only person who can determine whether you're Magnesium deficient.

If you want to go 'totally natural', here's a list of the foods you need to lean towards that are naturally high in Magnesium...

Nuts

Seeds (Sunflower, Chia, Sesame)

Lentils

Bananas and Dried Fruit (not too much as they're high in sugar)

Avocados

Brown Rice

Brown Spaghetti

Brown Bread

Wholemeal Bread

Dark Leafy Vegetables (Spinach, Kale)

Mung Beans

Kidney Beans

Cocoa Beans

Dark Chocolate 70-75% Cocoa, but only 1-2 pieces a day

Quinoa

Herbs are also high (per serving) in Magnesium are...

Thyme

Coriander

Basil

Dill

Spearmint

Another thing that might help you... Did you know that sleeping under a heavy blanket/duvet can help relieve Anxiety because the weight raises your levels of serotonin (the brain's feel good hormone) and this can improve your sleep? It's worth giving it a go. I tried it and I certainly slept much better and oddly enough, for longer.

Something that's also been known to help with anxiety is 'Mindfulness'. What is this exactly? The dictionary says that...

1) It's "the quality or state of being conscious or aware of something", and
2) "a mental state achieved by focusing one's awareness on the present moment, while calmly acknowledging and accepting one's feelings, thoughts, and bodily sensations, used as a therapeutic technique".

So, in short, it means you become aware of what's going on inside and outside yourself, as often as you choose to, including your thoughts!

If you start to feel anxious, try and make happy and positive thoughts the stronger and the negative and worrying ones the weaker. Your thoughts are SO POWERFUL, so be determined to enjoy the day with a smile on your face and see how well it works!

If you start your day with something that makes you smile, or even laugh is better, you'll instantly feel in a better mood and this lifts your spirits and quite often the whole day becomes better and better.

Save something on your phone that makes you laugh, smile or even dance so that it's always on hand when you need an instant boost. In fact, laughing and dancing is a brilliant way to help relieve Anxiety.

Now I'm repeating this, just in case you page flick and I don't want you to miss it. As we get menopausal and being anxious really doesn't help, one of the things that can happen is that your hair thins or falls out. It's because the follicle goes dormant, resting for a while and then starts growing again in a few weeks.

The problem with ageing, is that as we get older, the dormant period gets longer and the growing time of our hair gets shorter. So, more hair appears in the plug hole and your scalp gets more visible.

The speed of this can be down to genetics but either way, it's incredibly distressing and honestly, Anxiety doesn't help this at all and quite often, for a lot of women, the fact that they might be losing their hair, causes their Anxiety level to raise and it becomes a vicious circle.

Mine started falling out, you could see my scalp. I even started wearing a wig but, instead of just accepting it as part of the Menopause and getting even more stressed about it, I decided to see if I could find a natural remedy that would work and it did.

With incredible results!

In a few weeks my hair started to grow back and a few months on it was thicker and better than before and still is. The magic pill? Sea Kelp. I take 2 tablets daily in the morning and have never looked back. There's a lot of magic to be found in natural remedies, but more of that later.

The power of protein! Having protein in your diet releases the chemical serotonin in your brain, which can make you feel good help regulate your appetite and sleep. Boosting your serotonin is also widely used in medication to treat panic attacks, depression, Anxiety and phobias.

NOTES: What did you try? What worked for you? How long did it take?

8
Interlude - Time for a Giggle…

Before we get to the next chapter.

You know I said about losing hair on your head? Well, Mother Nature can be a bit cruel and some of us end up with hair where we don't want it. See if you can relate to this…

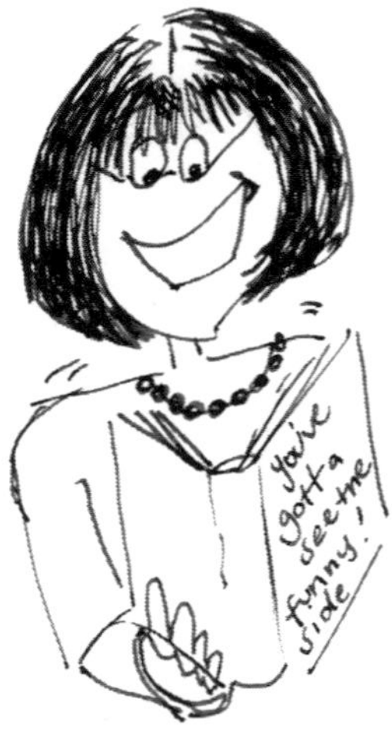

It was written by Fiona Loper and she kindly said I could share it with you.

"note to self:

when waxing eyebrows for the first time ever…

more is not better…

first of all…

<u>Step One</u>… warmer wax is good… however when it says microwave wax for 15 seconds… it's best to take note of actual time on the clock and not "GUESTIMATE"… I apparently am not spock… and I am guestimating my guestimate was off by at least fifteen seconds… but in my defence I was distracted by the cat walking past and farting… making my eyes water and my vision too blurry to accurately see the digital clock as those seconds counted down…

<u>Step Two</u>… applying warmed wax… I guestimate I skipped the part of the instructions that said… TEST THE TEMPERATURE of wax before applying in case you accidentally lather boiling napalm to your face…

<u>Step Three</u>… Step three occurs after the screaming stops and you have enough of

your wits left to attach the cloth strips to your face… having now effectively blind

folded yourself because you didn't have the foresight to think… "one at a time"…

<u>Step Four</u>… Grab the cloth strip and remove rapidly…There is nothing in the instructions to prepare yourself for this phase… There is no YouTube video of some middle aged menopausal loon attempting this for the first time…

And there is no warning about wearing hearing protection to prevent yourself from being deafened by the screaming noise that erupts at EXACTLY the same time as the cloth defoliates the mono brow shrubbery that has been clouding my vision…

and of course my impromptu screaming from the bathroom caused the sleeping dog to erupt in loud and sudden barking, which sent the previously napping cat into a fit of panic to leap without looking onto the safe refuge of the toilet seat… had I remembered to put the lid down… it would have been a safe refuge… which sent him leaping back out of the toilet, now wet and around my ankles.

Meanwhile I'm looking at my eyebrows… On the cloth strip…

I'm not panicking.

Judging by current rate of menopausally induced hair growth they will be back by tomorrow anyway…

I really need to send these manufacturers an email to add a few warnings to their product… for the stupid and inexperienced people like myself …

The only warning on the label was… DO NOT USE ON GENITALS

Really?... you have to WARN people not to apply napalm to their GENITALS? ...

Having read that I don't feel like quite the STUPIDEST person on the planet now."

I was crying with laughter when I read this and for me, this is what the menopause is all about. Having a sense of humour helps enormously and brings us all together and I actually had tears streaming down my face, as I obviously have a very vivid imagination and could see it all so clearly – or was it just that I could see myself doing exactly the same thing?!

9
Looking After You

As you get older, it's so important to really start looking after yourself.

Have you ever seen the quote by Patrick Flanery?

"Do Something Today That Your Future Self
Will Thank You For".

This is SO TRUE. Because whatever you do or start today, your future body and especially you will thank YOU for.

You have so much power over how you want to be, how you want to look. So that you LOVE what you see when you look in the mirror.

So where could you start?

Ok, let's start at the beginning... Get a nice mild exfoliator and rub it onto your face, neck, chest, arms and legs before you shower.

The menopause causes our skin to dry out and we lose that 'glow', so here's a few things that could help you...

Did you know that your skin renews itself every 27 days?

But thankfully not at the same time!

So get rid of those dead skin cells and see a new radiating you emerge.

You could try a natural exfoliator by using 1 teaspoon of Coconut Oil and 1 teaspoon of sugar, rubbed together in your hands so that it goes liquid and use that as an all over body scrub. It's so good for you as the Coconut Oil has natural healing properties as well, so is really great for your skin.

But what if you suffer from itchy/prickly skin? Try this... get a pot of Aqueous Cream to rub on, which is widely available, very inexpensive and can make a difference in just 2 days!

Is the skin on your face, neck and chest looking tired, dry or wrinkly? Again, THE magic product that has worked for me with INCREDIBLE results (e.g., wrinkles just about gone!) is 100% Pure Coconut Oil.

So, use it at night after you've thoroughly cleaned your skin, just a small amount as it goes a long way and using too much is unnecessary and can give you spots!

Massage it in and let your skin just soak it up and work its magic whilst you're asleep. You won't believe the difference it will make – and nor will your friends! I'll leave it to you as to whether you pass our secret on (wink).

Age Spots – seriously! Unfortunately, we all get them in varying degrees and sizes and these are often partly caused by extensive exposure to the sun, so it is massively important that you use Day Creams, Foundations/Tinted Moisturisers and especially Sun Creams with a good SPF factor protection in them, even in the winter.

Did you know that even when it's cloudy, UV light can penetrate glass and still damage your skin! It's the No.1 cause of premature skin ageing so the answer is whether inside or outside, to use

Sunscreen and Creams that have UV Protection in them (at least SPF 30) every day and help yourself look younger for longer!

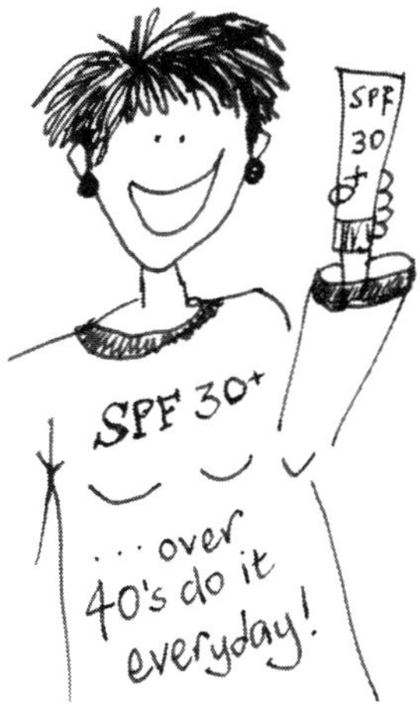

Another thing, if you have age spots that you might have and you want to try and get rid of them is Electrolysis. This is done over a matter of weeks by a qualified professional licensed electrolysis where they will treat the top dermal layer of the skin with an electrolysis probe.

A gossamer fine layer of skin is removed and often this is successful, but first the practitioner performs a sample test to determine if the age spot can be treated as sometimes the pigmentation of the age spot can go deeper into the skin which unfortunately means that there is no treatment currently at the moment.

If you have this procedure done and it's successful, you will be told to use a high factor, good quality SPF cream to prevent the age spot returning.

Unfortunately, Electrolysis didn't work for the age spot on my face, but where it was successful was with getting rid of a lot of my thread veins, both around my nose and on my legs, so maybe worth considering?

Or you could go back to good old nature again (which made a big difference to mine funnily enough) and use a cotton bud dipped in lemon juice and put it on your age spots, morning and night, after you've cleaned your skin and before your skin care routine. They honestly start to fade! And if you use Coconut Oil at night, this has been known to help fade them too.

As I said before, using a foundation or tinted moisturiser will help cover up any blemishes and age spots. This can work really well and helps give you the confidence that they're not noticeable when you go out, plus giving your skin protection when you do!

Unfortunately, for some women, thinning hair during the menopause is a devastating problem. Is your hair starting to thin or even fall out? DON'T DESPAIR – as I've told you before, (but just in case you haven't read this book, cover to cover) this started happening to me.

I can only comment from experience, (it was thinning to the point that I could see my scalp – I even took to wearing a wig!), but what worked and totally reversed it for me was taking 2 x Sea Kelp tablets every morning with breakfast.

I don't know how these tiny little natural tablets worked their magic, but they did and still do, because I still take them every morning. Be patient though. It took a few weeks, but I now have a full head of hair and it's even thicker than before! Oh – and it works on men too!!

Our daughters (in their 20's) also take it and their hairdressers always comment on how their hair is so healthy, shiny and how quickly it grows!

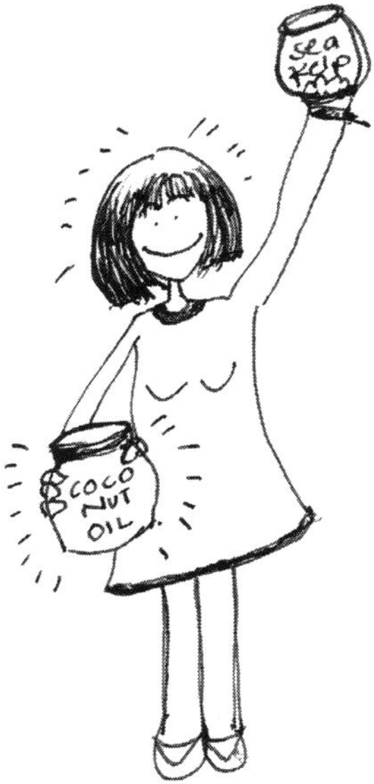

As you age, your teeth can look less shiny because the enamel wears down and you produce less saliva and generally we become more dehydrated (note to self - "drink more water"!).

One of the toothpastes I tried was Oral-B 3D White Pearl Shine and it really made a difference. It reacts with the surface enamel, coats it and makes it shine.

Another thing you can try is charcoal toothpaste which has a mild abrasion to it and that's meant to work wonders too, or you could just get natural charcoal capsules and empty them into a pot, then dip your toothbrush into it.

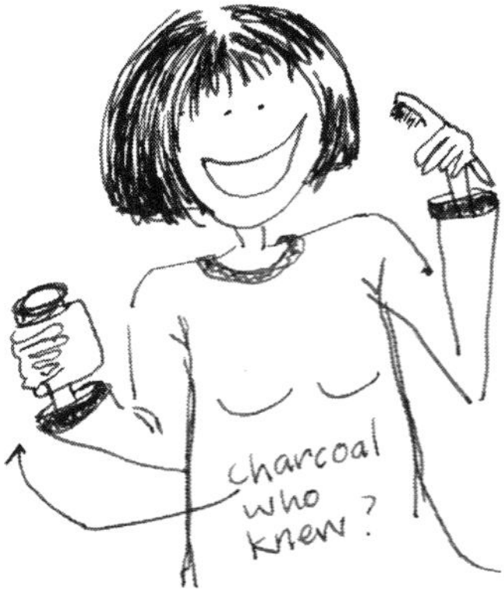

If you want to go back to Mother Nature again, then try this...

Mash a couple of strawberries into a paste and use with a normal toothbrush. The Malic Acid in them will help brighten your teeth, but you must always brush with a fluoride toothpaste immediately afterwards.

Try cutting back (or even out) tea and coffee as these stain your teeth, especially over a period of time, but when a woman I was working with tried this (and her teeth really weren't very white at all), I couldn't believe the difference in her when I next saw her! Her teeth were a completely different colour! I actually thought she'd had them lightened at the Dentist, but she told me that she'd just cut out tea and coffee!

The menopause can affect your hair, making it dry and/or dull. If this is happening to you, a small amount of 100% Coconut

Oil (here we go again!) makes a fantastic conditioner, (about a teaspoon size, depending on the length of your hair, so more if yours is longer) rubbed in the palm of your hands and smoothed through slightly towel dried hair. Work it from your scalp (works as a moisturiser) to the tip of hair.

Leave for a minute or so and then wash out with a small amount of shampoo. Dry as normal and see how shiny and soft your hair is! If your hair looks greasy after you've dried it, you just need to wash it out a bit more with shampoo, or not use as much oil next time.

Postmenopausal women are especially susceptible to dry-eye syndrome (due to a reduction in estrogen production) and your eyes can also sting, burn or feel scratchy.

To help this, get 'Hypromellose' which is known as 'artificial tears' and can be used safely to 'top up' your own tear level.

Don't get over the counter eye drops as your eyes can become very dependent on them and this will cause more problems! Wearing sunglasses outdoors will help too.

Now for a really 'bit of you time'...

So, generally, for a lot of us, Sunday is the 'day of rest' and I know us ladies don't often get half a day, let alone a day! So how about promise yourself an hour or more, later on today or one day or evening this week, to just spoil yourself with a lovely relaxing, warm bubble bath.

Accompanied of course with a class or cup of... (fill in your choice), some soft music, maybe a book, or magazine and just RELAX. You're special and you've not only earned it, you really DESERVE it and what a lovely way to end the week (sigh).

NOTE: Write down here, in order of preference, what you're going to try…

10
The Power of Positive Thoughts

Now I hope you don't think this is going to be 'heavy'. Please read on with an open mind and try and visualise the difference it could make to you.

Daily life can put such a strain on you, but coping with the menopause on top of that, means that you quite often feel like you're drowning. I know because I've felt like that, until I tried this and it really has made a difference.

I've put a few ways to go about it in this chapter as I hope one, if not more, will resonate with you and you'll be comfortable trying.

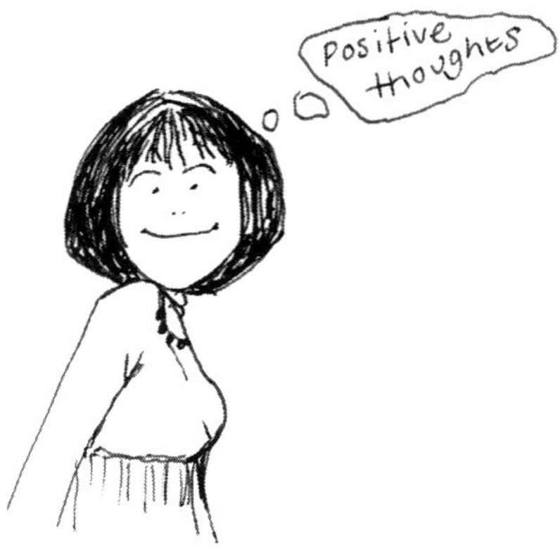

So, deep breath, here we go…

Remember – If you want to have a different result in your life, make a different choice!

You might not realise it, but YOU have the choice and power over your thoughts and what you do. The decisions you make are up to you and this will have a reflection on how your life will pan out, so think and choose wisely! If you don't think it's that powerful or even works – try it and see what happens, you might be surprised!

Another way to look at it is...

Remember that if 'Plan A' didn't work, you've got 25 more letters in the alphabet to go... so take the pressure off you because the right time and letter will come along.

Try and see the positive (wherever you can)

and seeing the good in things (if you want to)

and that happiness is a feeling you can have (in the choices you make).

Have you actually got anything to lose by giving it a go?

I say this, because did you know that if you make your thoughts positive at the beginning of the day, then it can literally change your whole day.

Because each day is a new day and a new start! So with that in mind, try doing this...

Don't think about tomorrow, because it isn't here yet. It will come, but not yet! So think about the NOW, what are you doing right now? What do you have to do right now? Concentrate on that, and only that and try and enjoy it as much as you possibly can. You'll be amazed at the difference it'll make, not only to you, not only to the rest of your day, but to how positive *you* become.

I tried this too, to actually test it and see what a difference it would make. Boy, was I in for a shock.

I wanted to write this book, but kept putting it off because it seemed so monumental. I mean, where do you start? So I did the 'NOW'.

I put everything else that I had to do out of my mind (the washing, ironing, cleaning etc., could all wait). I concentrated purely on the 'NOW' and with a blank, white new page facing me, I took a deep breath, sat up straight, relaxed and started writing.

Because I was only concentrating on the 'NOW'... I was enjoying myself so much that by the time I realised that I was getting tired, I'd written just under 20,000 words and had loved every minute of it!! Boy, do I love the 'NOW' and use it every day. All day if I can.

So, if you decide that you want to change your life where do you want to start?

What is the one area that would make the biggest impact on you?

Really focus on that one thing that you would want to change, hold that thought and vision strong and see if different and weird opportunities start to come your way – I've tried doing this and it honestly works!

Don't try to change your life overnight, just focus on making one change at a time and over time, all those small changes start to build up to BIG changes and your life starts to transform.

Don't give up because boundaries seem so constricting or unsurpassable. How do you know what you're capable of until you try? You might be pleasantly surprised how different your life could be if you stop saying "maybe" and start saying "yes"!

Ok, think of it another way... As I said before, who would you rather spend time with? Someone who looks as miserable as sin, or someone who looks happy and their face lights up when they meet you?

It can be as simple as changing the way you think, so start making positive steps to become the person you know people would like to spend time and have a laugh with.

Baby steps at first, easy to change steps like wearing a bit of makeup, or change your hair a bit, or make an effort with your clothes. Then build up to doing other things as your confidence grows – and it will.

Another thing that might focus you is to ask yourself, "I've got the rest of my life to live, so do I want to do it happy or sad?" Oddly enough, both take exactly the same amount of effort! (see below).

Stop 'wishing'. Just take a deep breath and start the journey towards the 'New You'.

Your thoughts really are that powerful.

It can start with an idea, like a hobby you'd like to have a go at,

a friend you haven't seen for ages that you could ring and meet up for coffee,

a poem that you'd like to try and write,

a 'she room' that you could make into your own haven.

It just starts with the 'start' - that first step.

There's a saying by Francesca Reigler (famous American Artist) who said

"Happiness is an attitude.
We either make ourselves miserable, or happy and strong.
The amount of work is the same."

Try and carry that thought around with you for a few days and see if it makes a difference, because if you are happier, then you have your own bit of magic for a better, more enjoyable day and future.

Ok, do this now, write down 5 things that would make a difference to your life, whatever jumps into your head is normally the right one to go for...

1) ....

2) ....

3) ....

4) ....

5) ....

Now were you smiling by the time you finished the 5th one? You see how powerful this can be?

So, now repeat each one out loud and *really* believe they will happen and let the magic begin. Because when you believe, you'll find that there's something amazing inside you, waiting to come out!

Look at something that makes you laugh, or play something that makes you dance and smile. This is really easy to do and quite instant!

Did you know that we ALL have beauty inside us? When things are sunny and bright for us we smile and glow and sparkle (a bit like when the sun shines through a stained glass window).

But it's when we are lit from within us, beneath our layers, in our heart, that's when our TRUE BEAUTY is revealed. It's always there, you can't see it until there's a break in our cloud and the sun streams through and transforms everything and everyone around us.

Sometimes you need a little help to make changes that will make all the difference, so maybe doing something like a new hobby with a friend.

Just know that making a difference is within all of us, but if you can work on making your life a happier one, one that suits you, then that's when you light up and your whole world changes, not just for you, but for everyone around you.

The other thing that might happen (and did to me), is that new friends will start to come into your life, ones that are drawn to the New You.

11
Practical Methods to Deal with Stress

I'm going to write a few things out that might help you and there might be some similarities with the last chapter because there is a strong connection between positive thinking and stress, and unfortunately there isn't a 'one size fits all' that will work.

You have to find the one that suits you, or maybe a few, depending on the time or what you're getting 'stressed' about.

So have a read through and hopefully you'll get some useful suggestions that will help. I really hope so.

These various suggestions have been known to really work for a lot of women who are buckling under the stresses of everyday life and then having to cope with the menopause on top as well!

They're here for you to try and get your life (and your symptoms) back into perspective and stop things overwhelming you - to take back control.

Keep reminding yourself that you can't change what happened yesterday, but you CAN change what happens TODAY and tomorrow hasn't arrived yet, so remind yourself not to stress about it.

Get a hypnotherapy CD, or download to your phone, lie down and listen to a calming voice, letting all your worries and stress just drift away and reduce the chaos in your mind – your face will relax too!

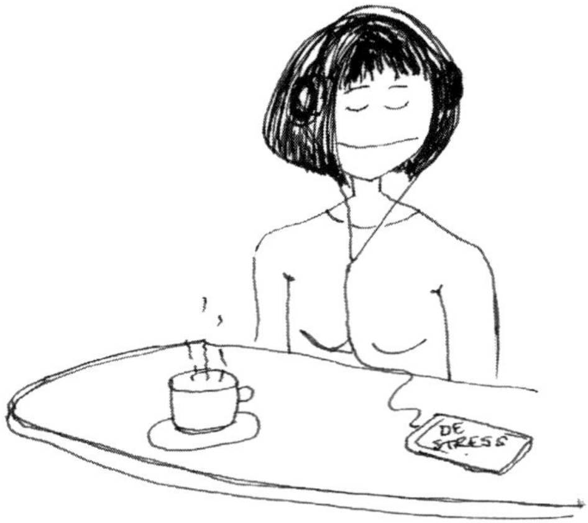

Try and stop things piling in on you because it's not good for you. Make a list for what needs to be done in 1 week, 1 month, then 3 months. Break it down, don't overthink things and by getting it out of your head, writing it down and taking things one week at a time, your confidence will grow and you'll be less stressed. It would be good if you could do this now...

<u>What needs to be done this week</u>

1) ....

2) ....

3) ....

4) ....

5) ....

What needs to be done next month

1) ....
2) ....
3) ....
4) ....
5) ....

What needs to be done by 3 months' time

1) ....
2) ....
3) ....
4) ....
5) ....

Now that it's all out of your head and you have your list, just tick them off when they're done. This will leave a lot more 'you' time to do the things that you really want to do.

I've been told that it's a fact that if you live in the NOW, you become calmer because you enjoy what you have, not what you don't! You can't change the past, so if you need to, try and learn what you can from it and let it go. What you CAN change is how you view today as it unfolds.

Find 5 things that you're glad of or makes you smile. Someone that you smile and say "hello" to smiles back at you? Is it enjoying the sun on your face? Or maybe treating yourself by doing something gentle like gardening, or baking, or sewing, or painting? Anything that's just for you and gives you pleasure. Write them down now.

The 5 things that make me smile

1) ....

2) ....

3) ....

4) ....

5) ....

We all have a 'To Do' list, so instead of stressing about how long it is, just choose up to 5 things to do today (or tomorrow if you're reading it later on in the day) – what are the *most important 3* that need to be done.

The top 3 things that have to be done by today/tomorrow

1) ....

2) ....

3) ....

4) ....

5) ....

The other 2 can wait until tomorrow. Spend the rest of the day/ evening on things that YOU really want to do, you'll end up feeling a lot happier and a lot less stressed! Try it, it works!

Ok, a smile moment...

Does anyone else have one of those days when you walk into a room and forget what you went in there for? Or go upstairs to get the thing that you've now forgotten and have to go all the way back downstairs and just stand there with a hopeful look on your face that you'll have a EUREKA moment?

Oh good. I thought it was just me! See… as annoying as it is, it's not just you going through it, so instead of getting stressed about it, smile and remind yourself of all your other 'sisters' experiencing exactly the same thing, and don't worry, because this stage will pass too.

What will help you and can do nothing but good, is eating 'brain' foods like…

Avocados	Egg Yolks	Beetroot	Blueberries
Rosemary	Walnuts	Salmon	Turmeric
Broccoli	Celery	Coconut Oil	Extra Virgin Olive Oil

Bone Broth (simple, cheap and easy to make)

Green Leafy Vegetables – Spinach, Kale, Swiss Chard and Romaine Lettuce

and the best one last…

Dark Chocolate (no less than 70% cocoa) YAY… But only up to 2 cubes a day (not bars!).

All these, incorporated into your healthy eating habits will not only help your brain, but can also have a positive effect on a lot of your symptoms.

Another thing that I found out was that relaxing is just as important to your health as exercising. Long hours working, looking after the family, endless lists of jobs to do, you really do need time to relax and calm, not only your body but your mind and stress levels as well.

So please allow yourself some 'relax time', just for you, every day, because it really is *that* important.

You could try Yoga. You don't need any equipment and you don't even have to go to classes if you don't want to. Just buy a DVD or take one out from your local library and put it on the TV, or just YouTube one and go through the exercises in the comfort of your own home, at a time to suit you.

You could even get a friend to come around and possibly have a giggle too, lifting your spirits even higher. It should only take about 15 minutes a day. Try and build up to doing it every day and see what a difference it makes to you. Not only will you learn to relax, you'll get stronger, it will definitely help your core muscles, will work wonders with your pelvic floor muscles and you'll definitely start to feel better in yourself. You really do deserve some ME time.

Laughter they say is the best medicine because it boosts your mood and lowers your stress levels. You really need to try this because it easy, free and you can do it on your own…

Go on YouTube and find things that make you laugh. Be warned though, it could become infectious and you might not be able to stop (what a shame). Just enjoy something for you, no explanation or excuse needed, just your laptop, iPad or phone. Oh, one more thing, you might want to go to the loo first!

What I'm going to tell you, I now do regularly because it really works for me and I'm killing two birds with one stone, so see if it works on you too!

Ok, picture this... I felt flat and to be honest, a bit fat as well (not good), so I had the house to myself, turned up the music, pulled my stomach muscles in (well, as far as they would go!) and danced from the top to the bottom of the house behind the vacuum cleaner.

Did I look daft? YES.

Did I get the housework done? YES.

Did I actually enjoy it? YES.

Did I feel like I'd had a workout? YES (my stomach still felt it the next day!).

Will I do it again? HECK YES (in fact regularly).

I smiled the whole time – brilliant!

Housework DONE.

Workout DONE

= one happy menopausal woman

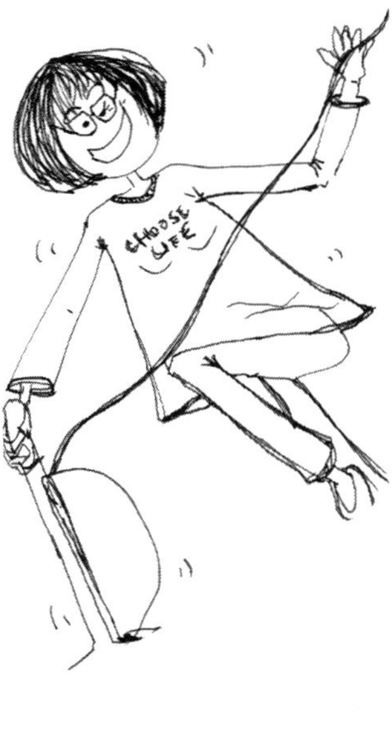

Ok, here's something completely different you could try, and you might not be expecting this but here goes…

KNITTING! Now don't dismiss this, as there are a lot of celebrities who knit (even men – like Russell Crowe) whilst on set to keep calm, relaxed and de-stressed so it must work! How does it work? It's due to the rhythmic and repetitive movements which promote the release of serotonin. It's claimed to…

alleviate stress and pain,

help with addictive behaviour

and can act as an anti-depressant!

It also acts as a fantastic boredom buster on a long journey.

All that with 2 needles and a ball of wool. Ok, if you can't fit them into your handbag, no problem. You could go 'mini' - get some children's knitting needles and download a poppy pattern, hats for premature babies in a soft wool (hospitals will love you), or a dog coat pattern and knit for a good cause wherever you go – everyone wins!

Another thing that has the same effect as that is 'hand fiddlers'. Easy to use and easy to store in your bag whenever you feel the need to just 'fiddle' at something.

How about breathing? No, I don't mean "but I do that all the time, otherwise I'd die" sort of breathing! To get rid of everything that's getting on top of you, try tuning into EVERYTHING that's going through your mind. Good and Bad… let it all in….

Give yourself a minute and then focus on your breathing. JUST your breathing and nothing else. Every part of the air going in, which organs use it? (nose, lungs, stomach, chest). You are now in control of your entire body, so realise that you can also be in control of your mind! It's yours, no-one else's and it's up to you to allow what you want in and out – like a breath, you can control it.

You have the power to allow positive or negative thoughts to enter your mind, just the same as you can decide to take a shallow or deep breath. Make your cup half full instead of half empty and see how much your life changes. This has been known to really work for a lot of women who are buckling under the stresses of everyday life and then having to cope with the menopause on top as well!

Someone told me they'd signed up to sing in a choir because it's been identified as one of the top 10 mood boosters (hard to believe - but even better than shopping!). Plus, they made new friends and had fun making a load of noise together. Oh, and a bit of a bonus – they were also boosting the proteins that their immune system needed to fight off illness at the same time!! Now that's one worth considering.

NOTE: Write down the things you've tried and the effect they had on you...

12
Find Your Fitness Potential

Now let's be honest with ourselves... We can be our own worst enemy and upping our fitness as we get older, will become our absolute best friend.

Here's a little test for you... Did you know that fit, 53-year-old women who can raise, from a chair, from a sitting position 53 times a minute without using their hands (have them stretched up for the ceiling, above your head), live longer?

I gave it a go and boy, could I feel it in the tops of my legs (a good thing no matter what the time of year as my trousers could look less like tights!) and my heart rate went up a bit too (it's a really good thing to exercise your heart and make it stronger).

Do it in your lunch break or as often as you want – the more you do it, the stronger and fitter you'll get. Plus, it doesn't need any equipment or cost anything! In fact, if you work with other people, do it daily to some music if you can and turn it into a competition and have a bit of a giggle in the office. Maybe even get the men involved – that could be interesting, who's the fitter, men or women?

Now how much fun do you want to have whilst getting fitter? Try Zumba. Honestly... not only will you get fit, you'll shed pounds (kilos) and can even reverse type 2 diabetes! Oh, and it also includes laughing and making friends. WOW, try suffering that once a week!

I read in a newspaper a while ago that menopausal women who did 2½ hours of fast walking or 1¼ hours jogging or running a week, plus strength or balance training (such as yoga) twice a week, were less likely to report anxiety, depression, memory and concentration problems and hot flushes! Exercise will also help you control your weight at a time when hormones are conspiring to pile the fat around your middle.

Walking is not only good for you, it's a way of pressing the 'pause' button for a while. Dress according to the weather and do this just for you. Your muscles, organs, hair, skin will all love you for it. You'll have time to think, to put things into perspective and order and when you ache a bit the next morning, you'll realise you're getting fitter too!

Promise yourself that you'll do it for 2 weeks (no matter what the weather). Because you'll start to lose weight, your fitness levels will go up, and as I said, your skin and hair will look better, your eyes will shine AND you'll see how quickly you begin to feel starting your day in a happy ready to go mood. People will want to know what your secret is!

You could start wearing something like a pedometer or fit watch which will also encourage you and is a gentle reminder, every day, to move more. Or use the free 'activity app' on your phone which (if with you) monitors how many flights of stairs you have climbed, how many steps you have taken and your walking + running distance.

Go to a 'ladies only' gym, which is a lot less stressful for you, you'll make friends and there's fantastic support on hand, whenever you're there.

This is all the more important because being overweight can exacerbate menopausal symptoms. It's definitely something worth considering incorporating some form of exercise into your week as much as possible as we all want to not only look but feel good too. Especially as we get older!

NOTE: Write here what you are going to try and then the results it gave you…

13
Brain Fitness

Sometimes the menopause can start to make you feel really down and low. Your body and mood seems to be changing all the time and you could feel overwhelmed with it all. It's been said that if you fill up your senses, this can push pain, depression and anxiety out of your mind.

Instead of your mind being full of thoughts and worries swirling around like a mixer, try instead filling your senses with being Mindful?

Bear with me on this one... Mindfulness is simply immersing and losing yourself in the joy of the moment. Like listening to nature, a soft piece of music, your breathing, looking at a beautiful view etc. It's allowing yourself some time each day to relax and recover from your daily pressures, a bit of down time that you can have/take, whenever you want.

Something that really helped me start turning my life around was when a friend said to me (after I'd had a good moan) "you do know that there's no such thing as the right moment, there's only NOW, so what's your excuse for not trying to change things? How much more time do you want to waste?"

That realisation was so powerful that I started making changes by changing my 'mind set' to "I can" rather than "I can't" and things, good things started to happen. So changing your mind set really can be life changing!

So get out of your comfort zone a bit because it's never too late and guess what, it gets more fun as you get older and you might discover a passion for something that you never even thought was possible.

Google evening or day classes and see if there's anything that interests you and write them down, that'll push you a bit. Yesterday's gone, but today is all yours, so enjoy it and be happy.

The 3 things that interest me as a day/evening class.

1) ....

2) ....

3) ....

Do you realise how powerful your mental state is to be able to give you the determination to get yourself out of a rut? Like your size, your mood?

Start walking everywhere to try and clear your mind, it's a fantastic mood lifter (it's been known to be one of the best tools to become happy) and also helps with self-confidence, plus the fact that it costs nothing.

All it takes is getting out of bed 15 minutes early, go for a brisk 10-minute walk around the block or around the field where people are walking their dogs already. Totally clear your mind and start to see the huge difference you'll feel. Or meet up with a friend or two. In fact, doing this, you might end up *with* a friend or two.

On top of that, doing as much as you can to keep your memory sharp is always a good thing, because our brains peak in our 20's and our memory starts to decline in our 40's.

By doing things like brain teaser games, crosswords, anything in fact that gets those little grey cells working, can only do you good and someone told me that tests have shown that doing these sorts of things, for just 6 months, significantly boosted brainpower in people aged 50+.

It's something that you have complete control over, to do as little or as much as you want, anywhere you want, as there are some fantastic downloadable apps for your phone or iPad. Or carry one of those sensibly sized travel crossword/word search style booklets around in your handbag and complete one page, whilst you're having a tea or coffee or waiting for someone.

Keeping your brain younger for longer is always a good thing and it's been said, can possibly help you reduce the risk of dementia.

Or maybe try this... if you're relaxing with a drink at home, try colouring in a colouring book as it's widely known that they're a great way to calm your thoughts, de-stressing you and nearly as good as meditating! So just have a bit of 'you' time and start colouring yourself calm.

On a more powerful note, have you ever noticed that the people who don't actually 'retire' look much younger than their actual age? It's because they're loving what they do, they're using their brains and developing their skills every day. This has a huge knock-on effect as to how they age!

It's honestly never too late.

Ok, the 'me' bit which will hopefully get you thinking...

How do I know? Because I'm 'talking' to you here, now. Have I ever written a book before? No! But I have now and I've also started a new career helping menopausal women worldwide look good and feel fantastic via a free Webinar giving all sorts of tips and advice, with a Menopause Help Programme, broken down into steps that can be done from the comfort of your own home, no matter which country you live in.

Did I know about any of this?

No. I've never used Facebook, Instagram or even knew what social media was, let alone how to communicate on it! But now I have thousands of followers from all over the world, regularly do Facebook lives, YouTube, and who knows what else will come along and I've done it in under 2 years, from scratch, aged 58 and really, really loving it.

So if I can do it, trust me, you can do it, if you want to.

Don't get me wrong, it scared the pants off me because it was like learning a completely new language and skill, starting from scratch, with stuff that I knew absolutely nothing about.

But if I didn't try to do this, would I regret it? Oh heck, YES I would, because at my age, what was I going to do with the rest of my life?

Now remember what I said about playing safe and saying "no", try saying "yes" and see where it takes you, and that's exactly what I did. I took a deep breath and said "yes", because there's always someone out there that can and will help you.

YOU'RE NEVER TOO OLD, so don't let ANYONE tell you that you are. You can do whatever you want, at whatever age, as long as you're not hurting or embarrassing yourself or someone else – JUST GO FOR IT.

I have, and what's really surprised me is how life is just getting better and better. I can feel my mind opening up (and I'm not the brightest button in the box) and expanding as each new challenge is conquered and my confidence grows.

I can't begin to tell you what that feels like (especially at my age), and I think that's what makes it even more special, until you try, or, if you're already doing something similar for yourself, then you'll know.

You don't need to do anything like this if it's not your sort of thing. We're all different and there are no rules. Maybe, just from doing something at night school might take your life in a totally different direction like doing something for craft fayres. It'll get you out of the house, earn you some money and could even get you travelling around the country to other craft fayres.

It could be anything, but can you see how your age doesn't need to be an excuse or get in the way of the dreams you have.

For example, I recently went on a Facebook course to keep expanding my knowledge and there was an amazing man there, soaking everything up, taking loads of notes, looking as happy as anything, constantly putting his hand up, we absolutely fell in love with him. He was 84!

14
The Power of Paws

How Animals Can Benefit your Life

Now I bet you didn't think that this would creep up in a book about menopause, but honestly, the health benefits of having a pet are HUGE.

They're not just your best friends, because cats also help with stress and loneliness.

Dogs not only do that, but also encourage you to get outside in the fresh air and exercise and this also opens up the opportunities of social conversations with the people who are also walking their dogs.

So how would you go about getting a pet if you don't already have one?

Funnily enough, it's easier than you think. You can just go to your local animal shelter, because there's most probably a pet there who is already waiting for you!

For some of us, the menopause can be a really lonely or sad stage of our life. Quite often the family has grown up and don't need you as much, or maybe your relationship isn't the same as it used to be.

Boredom sets in and this all has a huge effect on how you view life and getting older.

Well this book is all about the positive of the menopause and getting older, not the negative. So the benefits of having a pet is not only about the unconditional love that they give you, but the huge wellness boost that you'll get from it.

It's been well documented that having a pet (I don't think a goldfish counts) can decrease your stress, anxiety and even depression levels.

Doctors have also said that a pet can lower your blood pressure, decrease your risk of a stroke or heart attack and even (I remember reading somewhere) improve your immunity, so your trips to the doctor or feeling unwell get less and less!

Now is this starting to appeal to you?

What if you can't have a pet? No problem. Volunteer to help out at your local animal rescue centre and be the one that's there to help the wee things when they come in, bemused, scared and frightened.

How rewarding would it be to calm them down, nurture them and then see them go to a good home and a happy life? Talk about a win for you, a win for the animal and a win for the new family who's looking for that special 'pet' that you've had a hand in being able to now offer them.

No two days would be the same and the staff that run and volunteer in these places are incredibly special people, so you'll fit right in and also make some fantastic friends too.

If you prefer bigger animals, like horses and donkeys, then see if there are any animal sanctuaries near you, as they would love some help and the animals would love your attention too!

Maybe consider giving it a go, because you'll end up having a load of laughs too and how lovely is that? Plus, the animals you help nurture will really look forward to seeing you, as you are starting to teach them to trust again, helping them get ready for their new home and family. How special would that make you feel? Added to the friendships that you forge with the people who you work with.

15
You Are What You Eat – Literally!

When you begin the menopause journey, it starts to slow everything down a bit, and that includes how we digest our food, because it's not the same as when we were younger. So is there anything you can do about it now and does it mean going on another dreaded diet?

No, it doesn't and you might be surprised at some of these tried and tested suggestions...

Chew! It can be as simple as that. Did you know that it takes 20 minutes before your stomach even realises that you've eaten anything? If you swallow partly chewed food it's even worse, as it takes ages for that to get broken down, making you feel bloated, pass wind (charming), burp (lovely) or even have acid reflux!

The ANSWER... chew each mouthful 20-30 times, which means you'll eat less because you'll feel fuller sooner (because you will be) and your stomach won't have to stretch to accommodate that partly chewed food you swallow. Try it for 5 days and see the difference it makes.

We're increasingly told to cut down on the amount we eat, so try doing the following to make this easier. Did you know that we eat with our eyes first?

Serve exactly the same amount of food up on 2 plates, but put one portion on a bigger plate and the other portion on a smaller plate. Both these plates will have exactly the same amount of food on them, but your eyes will automatically tell your brain that there's more food on the smaller plate, than on the larger plate.

Try doing this for 1 week. Serve your meals up on a smaller plate and just chew (like I said above). I'll bet, by the time you get towards finishing what's on your plate, you'll be full. That makes it easier to start slowly cutting down on portion sizes and allowing your stomach to naturally get back to a smaller size.

The menopause can also affect your metabolism, so if you're feeling hungry, drink a glass of water first, because the chances are, your body is trying to tell you it needs water.

Did you know that our body is made up of about 70% water and that's why often we get hunger signals mixed up with thirst?

The other need for plenty of water is that dehydration can affect our nervous system, which triggers hot flushes!

Not only that, because your body requires so much water daily, if you make a conscious effort to drink more water and keep upping the amount you drink each day, not only will your body love you, your skin will love you too.

What I mean with this is that you'll visibly notice a difference, especially in your face because you'll be re-hydrating your skin and softening your wrinkles.

Oddly enough, drinking more water can also have a huge effect on reducing the bags under your eyes too.

Do you feel tired a lot of the time? If you want instant energy, then carry a small bag of nuts or seeds in your handbag. They contain high levels of Omega 3 and Omega 6 which are essential to your body, especially during the menopause. If you're allergic to nuts, then oat bars and whole grains work really well to boost energy too.

With the menopause, LDL cholesterol or "bad" cholesterol tends to increase, while HDL, or "good" cholesterol declines or remains the same, so if you want to significantly lower your cholesterol levels, fall in love with walnuts by nibbling 2oz a day for 6 months. Not, only that, they're also brilliant for your brain and nervous system too!

I know the menopause is something that we all have to deal with, but did you know that ageing is actually a matter of choice?

It's because a healthy lifestyle can slow or reverse many conditions that we associate with getting older like joint stiffness, type 2 diabetes, heart disease and more.

Hopefully that's enough motivation to start making changes that you can stick to, like drinking half a pint to a pint of water before each meal. Not only will you eat less (because you'll feel fuller), as I said before, water is essential to your body, skin and hair. Just making this one change can make a really big difference.

You could also try this, because research by Imperial College has found that "3 daily servings of wholegrains can reduce heart disease risk by 19% and diabetes by 51%, plus the added benefit of some fresh fruit and natural yoghurt". Now that's worth considering.

One thing you might not know, is that as we get older, our bodies develop an intolerance to wheat. It's because our stomach can't digest it well so it just sits there, around our stomach area, fermenting!! Try eating Gluten Free products, there's an ever widening range to choose from, like bread, pasta, couscous, biscuits, crackers etc., and you'll find it in the 'free from' isle in larger supermarkets. You'll feel so much less bloated if you do, as your body will be able to digest it more easily.

Now I know I'm repeating this, but it's relevant in this chapter too. Having protein in your diet releases the chemical serotonin in your brain, which can make you feel good and helps regulate your appetite and sleep.

It must be true because boosting serotonin is also widely used in medication to treat panic attacks, depression, anxiety and phobias.

Also, you don't need this book to tell you what a healthy 'diet' is, because if you're honest with yourself you already know which foods are going to be good for you and which ones are going to possibly see your weight creep up. So it really is up to you whether you want to go with the advice for a longer and healthier life...

It's not a diet at all, it just called the 'Mediterranean Diet' (mainly brightly coloured food) which means eating the sorts of food which will give your body all the things that it needs to be happy and healthy. It's as simple as that and one that a lot of women are considering as they are getting older.

Remember the saying... *"Do Something Today That Your Future Self Will Thank You For"* and your body works a lot more efficiently and lasts longer if you fill it with healthier things.

NOTE: The changes I promise I'm going to make to and for myself…

16
How to Love Your Body

The menopause, along with ageing, causes us to lose muscle mass, whilst our fat increases. This means that the two are out of sync and causes our body to store calories because it can't get rid of it like it used to - so we start to put on weight.

The long and the short of it is, if you continue to eat as you always have, but don't increase your level of physical activity, then it's more than likely that you're going to put on weight!

There's also a risk, if you start gaining weight after the menopause, that this excess weight can increase your risk of heart disease, type 2 diabetes, breathing problems and unfortunately various types of cancer including colon, endometrial and breast cancer. But, before you start getting worried, it doesn't have to be like that!

So instead of just giving in to the belief that every woman gains weight as she gets older – reverse this as much as you can by doing all the things that will make a difference in the way your body talks to you (lessening pain) and moves for you by...

Exercising (move more)

Eating healthily (so less of the rubbish and start re-training your body and mind).

Cut down on sugary food, drinks and sugar in your tea of coffee (use honey instead).

Support (from your family and friends for a better lifestyle – or even better, do all or some of this together!).

Cut down on your Alcohol as there's HUGE amounts of calories in these. For example, just in case you didn't know…

5oz glass of Red Wine	= about 125 calories
5oz glass of White Wine	= about 115 calories
1.5oz shot of Gin or Vodka	= about 100 calories
1.5oz shot of Whisky or Rum	= about 100 calories
1.5oz shot of Tequila	= about 100 calories
Bottle of Beer	= ranges from 64 calories to a huge 198 calories
Pint of Lager	= about 180 calories

This part you might not want to do, but will possibly be the best thing you do and that's to write down, and be honest (no-one else will see because it's *your* journal) exactly how many glasses of alcohol you consume on each day and then tot it up into how many calories you're taking in.

I'll give you a really good tip as to how easy it is to cut down, but for this first week, be as normal and then put an alarm in your phone for 1 month from today and do exactly the same exercise and see how much you've been able to cut down your intake (and possibly how much weight you've lost), just in that 1 month…

	This week		4 Weeks	
Monday	...... Glasses =	...... Calories	...... Glasses =	...... Calories
Tuesday	...... Glasses =	...... Calories	...... Glasses =	...... Calories
Wednesday	...... Glasses =	...... Calories	...... Glasses =	...... Calories
Thursday	...... Glasses =	...... Calories	...... Glasses =	...... Calories
Friday	...... Glasses =	...... Calories	...... Glasses =	...... Calories
Saturday	...... Glasses =	...... Calories	...... Glasses =	...... Calories
Sunday	...... Glasses =	...... Calories	...... Glasses =	...... Calories

Tip: after week one, put an elastic band on your wrist and as soon as you think you want another sip/glass, pull the elastic band so it 'snaps' on your wrist to remind yourself "NO" (this time have a sip/glass of iced water instead). It really works and you're now in control of how much you drink, rather than it being the other way around.

Ok, enough of the heavy stuff, here are some more ideas for you and your body...

Want to know a great way to make your waist smaller? It's called the 'Waist Whittler', burns over 200 calories in 30 minutes and works on your core muscles AND strengthens your pelvic floor muscles (a MUST as we get older)!

It's a hula hoop... get a large one (the bigger the better), or one that's weighted (they're not expensive) as this will give you maximum results and just persevere using it. If you're new to this, watch a YouTube hula hooping demonstration and you'll honestly, soon get the hang of it and a smaller waist is just the start of the difference you'll see in your body.

Just 10 minutes a day hula hooping can help get rid of that annoying weight we seem to have downloaded around our middle!

It'll also help with strengthening your core (stronger stomach muscles can give you a flatter stomach), strengthen our pelvic floor (bliss), burns calories (even better) and can be done at home even whilst watching TV, or out in your back garden just enjoying a bit of nature for a while.

All this with a circle! Then enjoy every minute of the admiring glances you'll get from friends and family as a cute waist starts to emerge.

Or even invest (not expensive) in a mini trampoline that you can put in the middle of the living room floor and bounce up and down on, whilst watching a TV show, listening to the radio, or getting into the zone whilst listening to a music channel.

Ok, if you think that's a little bit too adventurous, or you might be a little too 'old' for it (I doubt it though because all it takes is practice), then try a brisk 15 minute walk a day, because it's said that even if you're over 60 years of age, doing this can increase your longevity by more than 20%.

So imagine what it could do for you if you started younger than that?

Maybe even start a walking club? This is a fantastic way to meet other people and get fitter at the same time, plus it's known to make you happier. Oddly enough, it'll lead to other things like meeting up at the cinema for a night out together. That's exactly what happened to me and I've met the most wonderful women doing this, who have now become lovely friends.

Did you know that gardening can be good for you too? It's because you get endorphins from the actual movement of gardening (digging and weeding) and this helps block out your sense of pain and helps induce sensations of pleasure, like working with nature and hearing the birds singing.

It's also because daylight triggers a release of your mood–boosting chemical serotonin, as well as being a natural source of Vitamin D (assuming you're wearing sunscreen so you don't burn!). Not only that, it's lovely doing something for you.

Producing something that you've actually done yourself, by cooking those vegetables and herbs that you've nurtured, or arranging those amazing flowers that you've grown. You don't need to have a big space, use netting on a fence, hanging baskets, pots or tubs with compost in, or an edging to paving or pathways.

Use your imagination and just enjoy. Look at your garden as a 'room' and decorate it using plants of various colours, or go for a colour pallet and research all the plants you could have in your garden, of the colours you've chosen, to give you as near as you can, all-year-around flowering.

You can go to car boot sales and buy up cheap pots or containers and paint them to go outside to show off some of your new plants.

I was told that by doing it this way, planting your garden won't be expensive, as you'll buy the plants that are flowering at that moment for colour (where you have gaps in your garden) and then look for the ones that are flowering as the seasons change. Have fun making it into *your room*, a place to sit out in, with a cold drink in the summer and a lovely hot drink, wrapped up with a blanket in the colder months and just watch nature enjoying it as much as you are.

As you now know, the menopause and ageing is working against us with slowing things down, so we need to FIGHT IT...

So, if you want to burn calories fast – go to a dance class. You'll be happy to know that it burns more calories per hour than running, swimming or cycling. It's sociable and because you're having a bit of a laugh, you'll work harder without realising it.

There'll be a beginner's dance class near you so don't worry about standing out. Maybe get a friend to go along too, you can both have a laugh and get fit at the same time. What could be better?

Again water. Now I know I keep mentioning it, but it really is important. Hopefully you now know that up to 70% of your body is made up of water and that drinking water is so important for everything from your brain function to plumping out your skin (an absolute *must* during and after the menopause).

To find out how much you personally need to drink every day... divide your weight (in kilos) by 30 = the number of litres you need to drink each day (by the way, tea and coffee don't count, but hot water and fruit teas do).

Add different juices, mint leaves, sliced fruit etc., to make it more interesting for you. Measure out and put in the fridge your daily amount and then keep filling a nice, pretty glass and sip throughout the day and definitely drink a glass before eating any of your meals. This means that not only will you eat less, your bladder will get stronger and your skin, eyes and hair will start to look better. Again, people will want to know what your secret is.

Something I want to share with you that I found really interesting was that drinking cold water rather than room temperature water actually burns calories! One 16oz glass of cold water can burn up to 17.5 calories because you've drunk cold or even better, iced water, your body now has to work to raise its temperature back up to 98.6 degrees Fahrenheit.

Now that's *got* to be the easiest way to start losing weight and is something your body will absolutely love you for. Oh, and you might want to know another thing that will happen if you up your water intake to 4 litres plus a day...

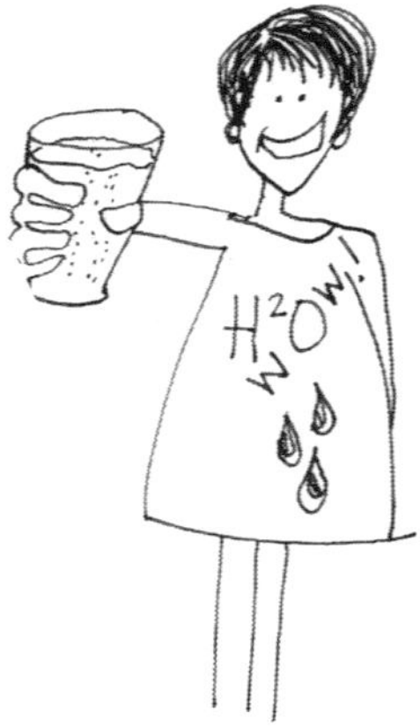

Your cellulite will start to diminish! We all know that water is essential to life and it's also essential to reducing and preventing further cellulite and that dehydrated skin looks shriveled, lumpy and old, whereas drinking a lot more water a day will plump your skin out and lessen the signs of cellulite. Make sure that the *first* drink of the day is a big glass of cold/icy water and you're well on the way.

Then, just try and get into the routine (in the bath or shower) of vigorously rubbing any cellulite areas with a bobbly body massage brush which generally have bumps or nubs to help stimulate blood flow and break up the solidified fluids below the surface of your skin which will then be re-ingested by your body and naturally got rid of. Worth a try?

Want to look younger?

Instantly?

I thought this might get your attention, because it certainly got mine...

In fact, there's two things that will achieve this for you.

First... Stand tall. It can be as simple as that to take years off you! It'll make you look and feel slimmer and give you less back, neck and shoulder problems. Consciously try and 'soften' your neck (don't tense it) and think 'tall'...

Something that might help, is to imagine a piece of string running straight through you and being pulled up through the top of your head, pulling you straighter and taller. It might feel odd to start with, but persevere and re-train your body. How weird would it be if people ask "have you lost weight?", "oh and by the way, are you taller than I remember?"

Second... Go to a department store and get the right size bra for you. I'll bet (like me), you're wearing completely the wrong size, maybe (again like me), not only the back size (34", 36" 38" etc.,) but also the cup size (B, C, D, DD, E etc.,).

Finding out your 'proper' size and getting those 'twins' positioned where they should be (not where they've ended up), will make a HUGE difference not only to your body shape, but your confidence, like you've never known.

In fact, (again, like me) you might be bumping into lamp posts or people as you walk down the road because you keep looking at this 'new woman' that you now see reflected in the shop windows that you pass.

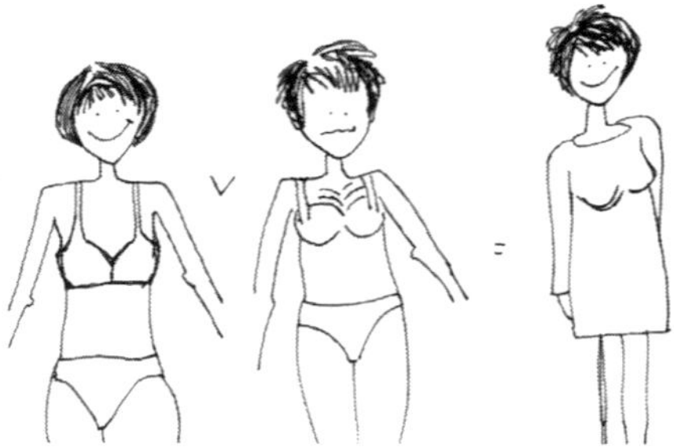

Another thing that your body wished you knew, but you can't see if it's happening is osteoporosis as it's one of those unseen problems that can occur with the menopause, but did you know that regular Yoga can help protect your bones (even if you've already been diagnosed with Osteoporosis)?

Plus, it helps fight off stress and makes you supple. There will definitely be a class near you and there are new people going all the time so don't worry if you've no one to go with, because by the next couple of classes you'll feel like you've know each other for ages.

It won't take you too long at all to be giggling afterwards seeing the positions you didn't know your body could get into! And if there are one or two women in the class that can wrap their legs around their neck – remember, they most probably couldn't do that before they started Yoga – so look how much more supple you'll get as you practice and the things that you could aim for!

Another thing that really helps with Osteoporosis, is standing on one leg!

Why?

Because standing on one leg for 3 minutes each day increases your bone density in that hip because of the additional weight bearing. I gave it a try whilst doing the ironing – boy did I feel it, but mostly in my bum! So double whammy – increased bone density and a firmer bottom – bring it on!

17
"But I Haven't Got a Thing to Wear!"

This is a longer chapter because for a lot of us, the way we look and feel in clothes can be a bit of a mine field and we all want to look good right?

So here, I talk about various things so that you can dip your toe in the water to start finding out what might suit you now and how to go about it and wherever you stick the pin in this chapter, I hope you learn something that will help.

So let's get going...

As I said before, the menopause and age has an effect on our body, so wearing flattering clothes can make a HUGE difference to your confidence! Just a good pair of jeans can make all the difference, worn with a shirt tucked in (accentuates your waist), or left out (takes the attention away from your waist).

If you've got good legs, then try skinny jeans with either flats or heels or boots. If you're not sure, then boot-cut is always a good option as they make your legs look longer and don't draw attention to any particular part. But make sure they cover your shoes and don't swing around your ankles, making it look like they've had an argument with your feet – not a good look!

Try and get as good a pair as you can afford, as they will last you ages, are never out of fashion and can be dressed up or down with a casual sweater, crisp white shirt or knock-out jewellery.

Did you know that fashion has no age limits? If you're bored with the way you look, you can change it and easily. I don't know if you're a bit like me and always played it safe with dark colours (black and navy being the favourite) and admired seeing women my age in lovely bright colours. But they look so good on them, but would most probably look a bit daft on me – boy was I wrong!

I was so fed up one day (I had the day off). It was actually when I was watching my normal early morning programme, that covers all sorts of topics to do with us ladies, including fashion etc., that I decided to go out.

I took myself off to a low budget store (just in case I got it wrong and didn't wear the clothes as much as I thought I would) and decided to be 'naughty' for the rest of the morning and pick things, totally out of my monochrome comfort zone. I could always take them back if I didn't like them when I got home.

I still kept my black and navy trousers but tried on bright tops with them. What a difference! I couldn't believe that my skin had more of a glow, so did my eyes and I actually smiled at my reflection – try it – it's AMAZING.

As I've said before, a good fitting bra is an instant confidence booster. Your clothes will look so much better on you and more good news – you'll also look younger! Your posture will improve and there is so much choice out there to help smooth your shape and make you look and feel great.

If you are a *Pear Shape* and want to get some trousers – (don't get them with pockets), try and get ones that are well cut and not tight so that the fabric strains. Hipster trousers will avoid the 'gaping waist' problem and will help to make your bottom look smaller! If you go for skirts, don't get them too short as this will accentuate your hips. Also, get necklines that focuses attention on your top half, like a cowl neck and a gilet to make your shoulders look wider.

If you're *Apple Shaped,* then opting for a wide, open neckline, will keep people's eyes away from your tummy. If you need to, invest in a push-up bra, and wear clothes that accentuate your waist with a belt or detail and again wear some knock-out jewellery.

If you're a *Straight Up and Down Shape,* invest in a push-up bra (if you need to) and opt for tops, patterns or belts that draw attention to your waist, so giving you a more 'womanly' figure. If you have a smaller bust, then you can get a control bra with chicken fillets, but remember, those twins don't need to be under your chin, as that is not a good look.

If you're an *Hourglass Shape* – oh lucky you, as this is meant to be the sexiest shape there is and has been since times long past! Your waist will look tiny because of your boobs and hips, so wear clothes that accentuate it for that really feminine look. Steer clear of frills though – just too much going on!

If you're a bit of a *Top Heavy Shape,* then, by all means, show a bit of cleavage (as this is your asset), but balance it out with wearing trousers or a skirt that makes your legs look amazingly long and with a heeled boot or fabulous shoes. If you're very tall, then get tops that give you a bit of a flare out around your hips, or that are gathered into the centre of your body to balance things out.

Now SHOES – (and this comes from a 'Shoe Queen'). The menopause can give us aches and pains and we all want to look good when we go out, but honestly, trying to totter around in heels that we used to be able to wear for hours on end, but only now seem to be suitable for looking elegant sat down (heaven forbid we need to get up and try and walk elegantly to go to the ladies) now has to have a total re-think.

Heels that are too high to walk comfortably in won't give you enough confidence when you walk into a room or dance! Smaller heels will improve the way you walk without the worry of twisting your ankle of killing your feet when you're twirling around a dance floor and remember comfort is key, but can be stylish too.

Sorting your wardrobe out can also have the most dramatic effect on you by getting rid of all those memories that you no longer want.

Because the menopause and general ageing will change your body shape, there will be clothes in there that you will honestly never wear again and trying to stuff yourself into your old clothes will never make you feel or look good. You need to take control and forge ahead with the new you.

Have fun discovering who you are. A bit like I mentioned above when I went shopping for a bit of a change of colour. You'll be amazed that what never suited you before, now does! It's because not only your shape, but your hair colour, even your skin tone has changed as you've aged, so look on this time as very liberating and a totally NEW CHAPTER. Have fun!

Declutter your wardrobe! It's unbelievably powerful. Ok, wardrobes, cupboards and drawers need to be gingerly opened and not just looked at and closed again (easy), but gone through and decisions made (harder).

Why should you do this? Because, honestly, getting rid of the clutter will make you breathe better because you'll only keep things that suit you, fits well and makes you look amazing.

Get rid of everything else because I bet you don't wear it and it staggered me how much I actually hadn't worn for ages, so that means you don't need it. It'll have the most amazing effect on you and a difference when you get up to get dressed in the morning, or have to decide what to wear when you go out in the evening or for a special occasion.

Because the one thing that surprised me the most, was that although I ended up with fewer clothes, I actually had more choice! It's because I'd got rid of all the things that had been bulking my wardrobe out, which meant that I couldn't see what I actually had that I could make outfits out of, if that makes sense.

For a lot of women, the menopause can cause your boobs to get bigger ("yippee" for some women / "you have got to be kidding!" for others).

As well as getting the right fitting bra (as I mentioned above), if your chest is getting larger, then a flattering shape for you is a wide V-neck that cuts from the edge of your shoulders. It gives the effect of lifting and separating, but also draws attention upwards towards your neck and face, without covering up your assets! Teamed with a great pair of trousers, jeans or skirt – you'll look amazing for any occasion.

Also, as I mentioned before, for a lot of us menopausal women, our body shape changes and looking good in some clothes – especially going out for a special evening or occasion can pose a problem because we have lumps and bumps where we really don't want them! We all need a little bit of help so don't despair because there is a solution...

Shapewear (Google this if you don't know what it is).

Now getting in and out of them can be a bit of a challenge! So here's a couple of tips...

Tip 1: Step into it and pull up gradually, releasing the fabric as you work up to the top.

Tip 2: Go for your true size, it will do the work it's meant to, rather than thinking a smaller size will make you look smaller. It won't because it'll end up being painful, riding up or down, or giving you unsightly bulges – not a good look and totally defeats the exercise in hand (which is to look as sexy as possible).

If you have a bit of a muffin top, go for high-waisted shapewear.

If you have a bit of wobble on your thighs, go for ones that look like long shorts.

If you are in need of a bit of all over coverage, then go for a body.

If you have a nice bum (lucky you) but a bit of a tummy, then they now do control pants that are shaped like a thong, with a large control panel area for your tummy.

You can get the ones that are particularly good at sculpting the waist. But for more comfort, get the ones that go to the top of your knees as a VPL (Visible Panty Line) isn't a good look!

Plus, you don't want to spend your whole time whilst you're out, trying to get your shapewear to where you had it when you first put it on. So choose wisely and for the areas that you need controlling the most.

Nobody else is going to see what's under your outfit (well hopefully) and if they are, that's not a problem. Wear some lovely looking (matching) underwear underneath and do one of those sexy, mysterious exits into the bathroom (you know, the ones that you see done countless times in the films) take your shapewear off and voila! Sorted.

When you're shopping for any clothes, please don't beat yourself up on dress sizes either - *all retailers size their clothes for a slightly different fit,* because there's no such thing as a standard dress size! Take a size, above and below what you think you are, in with you when trying on and don't even look at the number on the label, but by how it fits, feels and falls on your body.

Why? Because you know that when you look at your reflection in the mirror and absolutely love what you see, then it's like a pin popping a balloon when you look at the number of the size in the label, especially if it's a higher number than you were expecting. So please, DON'T DO IT.

You don't have the size on show so no-one needs to know what it is, so when you get home cut out the labels. They and you just need to see what you see in your reflection, a great looking woman, looking amazing in her new clothes.

Now, the only way that this absolutely turns itself on its head is if you're actively losing weight, or looking at is as inches is a better way. Then seeing the size numbers coming down is a fantastic morale booster and will definitely keep you on track and focused.

18
When Being Selfish is Good

Pleasure is a priority, not a treat and if I was working with you, this is one of the things I would be asking you about, each time we spoke.

It's so important to take time just for you, as constantly giving for everyone else and not taking time for yourself can drain the life force from you. Lose yourself in whatever feels right for you,

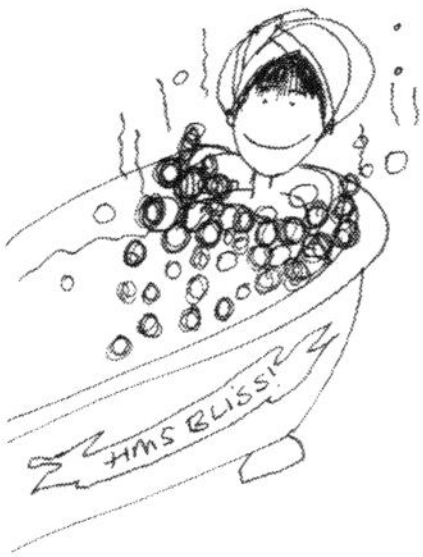

A warm bubble bath.

Watching a funny film.

Dinner or lunch with friends.

Doing your nails.

Experimenting with your hair.

Going to a show.

Dancing around your kitchen with some really good music on.

Watching a film that you love and has the real 'feel good factor' for you.

Relaxing and reading a good book or magazine with a scented candle lit…

A bit like I'm doing now, whilst I write this. I've got some lovely soft music on, a scented candle lit, it's just you, me and my lovely rescue cat curled up on the chair beside me and I'm loving every minute of it. Calm, relaxed, a smile on my face and just 'chatting' to you – bliss.

Do whatever nurtures your soul. Look at it as an essential health benefit.

Again, something just for you…

Having a good chat with friends and interacting with others can bring out a deep sense of relaxation and happiness for you. Did you know that talking triggers a flood of chemicals that scientists say gives women a 'rush' like a 'high'! No wonder us women like to talk!

Write down 7 things that you think would 'nurture your soul'. Some could be easy to do and a couple maybe more of a treat and that you'd love to do. But this is for you and what *you* want to do, so don't hold back, just go for it…

1) ....

2) ....

3) ....

4) ....

5) ....

6) ....

7) ....

19
How to Overcome "I've Got a Headache"!

Now you most probably knew that this was coming, but this chapter is focused on things from your partner's point of view.

You'll notice I didn't say the menopause from his point of view, that's because he most probably (and maybe even you) doesn't even realise that you're changing because of the menopause and this will affect both of you in one way or another.

Don't worry, there are more 'chapters' that will allow him to see it from your point of view and one that he (and possibly you) might find surprising, but more of that later.

As I mentioned earlier, loss of libido is a common menopausal symptom so you might become more withdrawn from your partner and they don't know how to help you as they don't understand...

what you're going through,

or even why,

or that you feel the way you do.

To be honest, you most probably don't really understand it yourself either and that's to be expected and is perfectly normal as (I don't know if you know this), our sex drive decreases gradually with age in both men and women - but women are two to three times more likely to be affected by a decline in their sex drive as they age.

But don't lose hope, because for the majority of women, after the menopause, everything gets back to normal and for a lot, even better than before (if you know what I mean).

You need to know at this point, that loss of sex drive or even desire is *far more common* than you could possibly imagine.

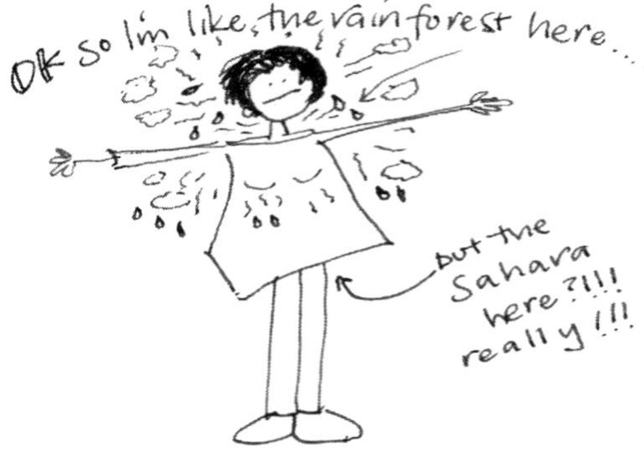
OK so I'm like the rain forest here....
but the Sahara here?!!! really!!!

But because nobody talks about it (most probably because you don't want to be seen as the only one "not getting it"), you keep quiet and get more and more wound up by it because you think there must be something really wrong with you.

Let me explain why this is most probably happening to you, and maybe this is one of the sections you wouldn't mind your partner reading as it could very well explain things to him. Don't worry, I'm not going to get graphical, but it's to try and tell you why you're possibly feeling this way.

So firstly, why is this happening to you? It's because the menopause causes falling estrogen levels, which one of the side effects is vaginal dryness and this can cause sex to be very painful.

Your testosterone (I actually didn't know us girls had testosterone) can start to reduce as well and this affects your 'desire' and for us women who have to have a full hysterectomy (ovaries removed as well), will cause you to have an immediate drop in both estrogen and testosterone and a greater increase in your lack of 'desire'.

This can cause frustrations, not only for you but for your partner as well, because it's something that can't be seen, so a lot of us just don't know why we're feeling, or not feeling like we used to, and because of this we do nothing but grow apart, not talking.

How on earth do you bring this sort of subject up, or even try and describe or talk about something you don't even understand? So you just start to close up.

He thinks you're going off him because you used to 'want it all the time' in his eyes and now you'd rather do anything but!

A physical touch is important, even the squeeze of a hand or an arm around the shoulder can make all the difference to a barrier being up or starting to be taken down in our relationship.

As we get older, it seems that us ladies are waiting for our partner to make a move, even a small one. As I said above, like the squeeze of our hand, or an arm around our shoulder or even something as simple as a "thank you" as a sign that they appreciate all that we do, every day, around the house, for the family, for them.

But unfortunately, stalemate can occur and men are particularly stubborn for making the first move, so, like with anything they don't understand or don't want to discuss, they just go back into their 'man cave' = subject closed, or not even opened to be honest!

Well, we ladies are so much stronger than that and sometimes, all it takes, is for the door to open slightly, so try this and see what happens...

Maybe start to break the ice first by sending a text to him, thanking him for the cup of tea he made you?

Now why a text? Because it's out of the norm and totally random, which means he's not expecting it AND he can keep it to re-read when he has a soft moment (and they all do).

There was magic there at the beginning of the relationship but there's something even nicer to have as we grow older and that's companionship and peace, with smiles and the touching and holding of hands.

Please don't think that this is how it's going to be from now on in – the odd touch of a hand, and then you both go off to get your slippers and sending each other a 'random' text now and again. It's honestly not like that.

This is just to give you an idea of how to keep the connection going between you and start the re-connection process, because after the menopause, when everything's settled down and finished, you should be right back to normal and the lights are green... In fact, for a lot of women, it's even better than before because no more periods, all risks of getting pregnant have gone and they've found it very liberating!

The other piece of advice I'd give you that could make all the difference in the world, is *talk* to your partner/husband.

Tell him what you're going through. I didn't say 'her' because, to be honest, she'll understand it because of puberty and periods, but just in case she doesn't, then read on. But unfortunately men *really don't* understand. That is...

Until they're told.

Until you spell it out.

Until you explain.

Have you any idea what it must be like to watch your partner/ wife change so much from the woman they fell in love with and not have a clue why she is now changing into someone he hardly recognises and can't talk to?

You most probably don't. He's scared, frightened and maybe for once in his proud life, he can't put it right. Because he doesn't know what the heck is wrong!

Maybe it's his fault?

Are you going off him?

Maybe you don't love him anymore?

Maybe you've got 'someone else'!

Maybe you're building up to ask him for a divorce (so into his 'man cave' he goes).

And on and on it goes, like a gathering snowball, getting bigger and bigger until he's convinced himself of something that is so far from the truth that it's laughable, but too much time (and snow!) has gathered and the barriers are all up and also because of the conclusions he's come to (all on his own), so how on earth do you start to break them down?

Suddenly there's a she-cat prowling around the house just waiting for her next prey.

She's angry at everything, anything. Even going completely off on one because she's seen a cobweb in the corner, or as Nancy said (which you'll read later), 'the butter was put in the wrong place in the fridge. Seriously'!

He doesn't know what to say because he doesn't understand, and oddly enough that makes matters worse, for both of you!

He most probably thinks you just don't fancy him anymore (and so the downward spiral starts) because you used to be intimate but he won't understand (until you tell him) that you've gone off sex and it's not his fault.

Possibly, that you daren't let him be in your airspace, just in case he wants to cuddle you, because you *"know what he's thinking"* and one thing will lead to another and, at the moment 'another' is the last thing you want!

If you explain how you feel, that it's not him that's the problem (men are just too proud), but that it's you, and that you'd love nothing more than a cuddle, but just a cuddle.

Maybe once in a while you'll go on a 'date night', get dressed up, enjoy each-others company and when you come home, you'll concentrate on him. He'll most probably be quite happy with that (they're simple souls a lot of them).

Actually, another way of looking at it (from his point of view)...

Remember I said before, that as we get older both men and women's desires can wane a bit? Well maybe his has as well, and he's scared to death that you've noticed and are 'cooling' towards him (because, honestly, men pin far too much importance on sex and think it's the 'be all and end all').

So then all the "maybe she's" that I mentioned above, are swirling around in his head and off he trots to his 'man cave' to sulk because there's absolutely no way that he's going to broach that subject. Absolutely not. NO – SERIOUSLY! - because men don't do that!

That's why we're known as the stronger sex. It's because we tend to tackle things and get them sorted, rather than bury them and hope that they'll go away – they rarely do! And, like anything buried, it festers, goes mouldy and rots. So it's best not to let it get to that stage.

It might even make it easier for you to explain if you show him the next chapter, because it should open the doors to communication between the two of you (or maybe even other members of your family that don't understand what you're going through).

He'll either fully understand a lot of your symptoms and maybe even point ones out that you don't actually have, but it makes him feel like he 'gets it'. So please don't have an argument, just love the fact that he's trying to help you and gently explain, how he can – even if it's just being patient.

Or he'll be absolutely flabbergasted and realise that it could be so much worse (for both of you) and he'd better just help you as much as he can. Just think, if a load of us women don't know what the heck is going on, how on earth is a man supposed to?

There's so many things that you can do to try and make this stage of your life easier. Not only for you, but for the whole family.

Not only that. If you understand one another, your future together has so much to look forward to because honestly, you will come out of this even stronger than before and you'll most probably, slowly, love being intimate again.

It'll be like the beginning all over again.

You just need him to understand.

If you need a bit more help with this complex subject, I don't know if you've read the book "Men are from Mars & Women are from Venus"? If you haven't, you really must, but someone (who knows about these things!) told me once that men and women communicate differently, so I'll tell you what she told me which really makes sense and is easier to understand and that is...

"Men speak to give information, women speak to create emotional bonds and we seem more capable of understanding and talking about our feelings, which gives us release so we don't bottle it all up.

Men put all their effort of emotions into actions – they don't talk!"

So maybe write him a letter, explaining your symptoms, emotions, feelings, worries about what you're going through. He can then take his time over this and really understand what bits are effecting you specifically and this will break down a lot of barriers and you'll be able to meet him half way and he'll know what to expect because you've already explained it to him. So no nasty, embarrassing conversations, just possibly, what can he do to help?

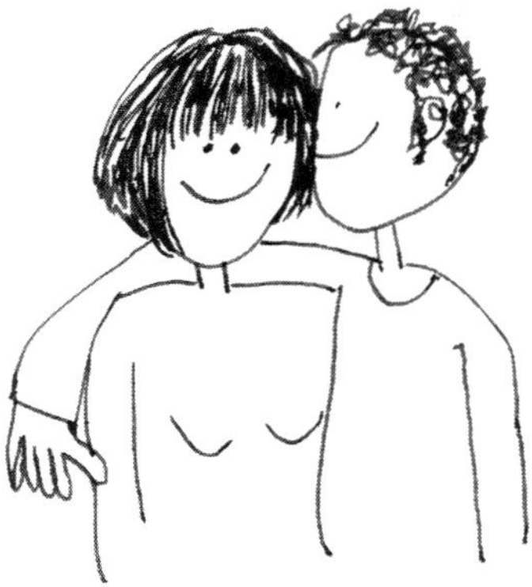

If you want him to start talking, you have to go slowly and be patient (Rome wasn't built in a day and all that), so when he does start talking LET HIM TALK!

Don't interrupt – *AT ALL*, remember – silence is golden! Because as soon as you start to talk, he'll shut up and you'll have to start all over again!

Just listen... Don't apportion any blame, try and keep your feelings to yourself (if you're feeling really menopausal, he just won't get it), just give constructive (easy peasy) feedback to keep the new line of communication open and him beginning to understand – like the rising of a new dawn, soft and gently does it.

Men aren't as complicated as we are and that's because they don't understand us, because that's what our girlfriends are there for, because they do!

But if we can make it easier for them just to talk, funnily enough it makes our lives easier too! It's worth a try, but be patient as the end result will hopefully be that calm we need and laughter is restored = a very happy woman, home and hopefully relationship.

NOTE: Write here what you're going to try and then tick it if it got the right results…

20
'The Menopause' from a Man's Point of View!

Now I know you weren't expecting this as a chapter so I'll tell you why I've put it in this book...

I hope, your partner might find this really interesting, especially if they don't understand what you're going through and its difficult for you to explain, or they think you're being dramatic and it's just 'women's problems' and switch off!

I think it's important for them to try and understand, in a man's opinion, what it's like to have hot flushes and abdominal pains/ cramps.

Now let me explain... This chapter has come from my husband (now get those raised eyebrows back down lol).

No, he hasn't had a sex change or anything drastic like that to enable him to be able to write on this topic. He has Prostrate Cancer and as soon as it was diagnosed and even before the Radiotherapy had started, he was put on a drug called Prostap 3, which is a female hormone, designed to supress all testosterone.

The side effect of this is that he gets hot flushes and abdominal pains (due to IBS from the Radiotherapy). He's had these for the duration of his treatment (four years at the point of writing), so he knows exactly what I'm going through and we often peg out the washing together to cool down at the same time.

So, from him, in his words – this is what it's like to have a hot flush from a man's point of view…

"HOT, HOT, seriously… HOT!!"

There you have it, from a man, explaining beautifully what it's like to have a hot flush!

I'm sorry, but this just will not do, so I'm going to have another attempt at him trying to explain in more than 4 words, what it's actually like.

So, bear with, I won't be a moment, a little word in his 'shell like' (ear) coming up. I told you men don't like to talk and it can be like trying to get blood out of a stone if you want them to, so here goes (maybe put the kettle on, I could be a while!)…

Well that worked! Ok… here we go…

"It didn't take long, after going on the injection for these "things" to start to happen – I couldn't believe how violent they are, how all-consuming they are in respect of their intensity and the fact that I have absolutely NO control over them whatsoever.

They come on, any time, any place, anywhere and sometimes are as frequent as 1 or 2 an hour! They can last about 1 minute, up to 5 minutes. You get no warning at all.

The only way I can describe it to you is that the feeling seems to start in my head – literally, my head gets hot and the sweat just runs down my face, it then progresses to my arms and hands, where again the sweat beads all over them, with a prickling sensation (like nettle stings) as the sweat forces its way out of my pores. It then spreads throughout my body, down my back and my legs get clammy! IT REALLY ISN'T FUNNY!

The only way I can think of you understanding the intensity of them, is to imagine that you're put fully clothed into a sauna and not allowed out! It makes no difference whether it's a hot or cold day, what you're wearing – NOTHING MAKES A DIFFERENCE, because it happens from the inside out. I have absolutely no control.

They are wearing, exhausting and to be honest, embarrassing as there's nothing I can do about it! I could stand in a fridge and it would make no difference at all – it would still feel like I was stood in a sauna and this happens both during the day and all through the night. And then afterwards – when they subside – your BLOODY FREEZING!

I have no idea how all these women can put up with them. I've tried natural remedies but nothing seems to work, maybe it's because I'm not a woman (thank God). I constantly have a flannel or towel with me, I had to start wearing a vest to try and soak up the sweat, so how ladies deal with them daily and at night, I have no idea at all. It's miserable, totally miserable.

My advice to you if your partner is going through this, is just be BLOODY UNDERSTANDING and thank your lucky stars that you're not going through it!

The abdominal pains aren't as frequent and were a by-product of the Radiotherapy (it's IBS). When I started to get them my wife gleefully crowed "that's just like a period pain, now you know what I've been going through all these years, every month, for a whole week at a time". For once, I actually didn't have an answer!

*I've had to really think about my advice to you on this subject and all I can say is its S***, honestly, it's S***.*

There's no way I'm coming back as a woman – SERIOUSLY!!

How on earth do they put up with pain like that? It's literally like being doubled over after being kicked in your gonads! The cramp feeling is so intense; I can't get rid of it. To say nothing of the urgency to get to the bathroom.

So if this is what it's like to have a period you can BLOODY KEEP IT (excuse the pun)!

You're getting an idea of how I feel because there's a lot of "bloody's" going on. Honestly guys, cut her a bit of slack, in fact, a LOT of slack.

How she deals with the menopause (and I've only experienced two of the symptoms that she could get), I have no idea, on top of running a home, and possibly you, and all the other things that I'm amazed that they do. Just be thoughtful, kind, loving and most of all, understanding.

She's not putting it on, she's just trying to deal with the menopause (which I'm told by my wife is like puberty in reverse) as well as she can (because she's hasn't got an option) and believe me, if you're fed up with it – think how she feels.

I just want to get my life back and can't wait for these symptoms to end.

THE END. Now I'm going for a lie down (I can't believe she made me do that!)".

Oh but I am!! Now that's *much* better than 4 words lol, bless him xxx

21
Sex and The Menopausal Woman!

Now I've done enough talking, so this was written for me by a lovely friend of mine, who's managed to keep her love life going, both her husband and herself happy and their relationship close and strong.

Sex and the Menopausal Woman

So here's the cheeky bit, yet it's often the profound bit if you're in a relationship. We've talked already about how confusing this change is for you.

Sometimes the menopausal symptoms creep up on you and you find yourself behaving in a way that's different, angrier, more frustrated and by golly, if each individual symptom took you a little bit by surprise, or took a while to show itself as a repeated behaviour, then this is why you're constantly a confusing ball of fury for him.

I found that anxiety, or anger, or tiredness, or weight (and therefore self-esteem) 'snook up' on me and until I took time to realise what was happening, I thought

"Oh, my God, that's it, we're falling apart, we're not connecting anymore"

I (obviously) reflected the whole problem on me...

"I'm dry",

"I'm really not feeling like it"'

"I can't spontaneously do it as we have teenagers in the house with acute hearing, simply listening out for Mum and Dad having sex – 'cos they've nothing better to do!"... and other such histrionics!

For a while I would avoid sex and the wonderful intimacy it can create in a relationship. Although it's not the be all and end all for lots of women, for a lot of men it is.

I came to realise I was avoiding any touch, just in case it led to sex. I was on shutdown mode... this was not good for my marriage of 24 years, which I value deeply. I love my husband and equally he loves me back (I feel very lucky that way), but it's a standing joke between my friends that his libido is hysterically high, compared to mine!! We're compatible in every other way possible, but that's our funny 'difference'.

Apart from all my other daft little nuggets of ideas about how to "get back in the game again", I must explain that once I made a determined effort to 'play' again, I realised, half way through, I would be thinking "oh, I'm totally into it now, we should do this more often" (I said in my head "he needs no further encouragement").

For me (and I by no means speak for all women), I find the intimacies that regular sex creates in our relationship is invaluable... I love being his best friend too, but I want more... More of what he can't get from anyone else... I'm his soul mate, not just a buddy.

Anyhow, after very frank discussions with female friends (I'm lucky I have some wonderfully 'filthy' friends and I mean this is in a fun, not demeaning way), we discussed all sorts over the months and even years about new tips, new products etc., etc.

I find the more open you are with friends, the better on this score

a) Because it sorts the wheat from the chaff – who are really "your people",

b) I found out lots of fabulous hints and tips,

c) I found out that everybody has "barren" times, and more importantly, that you can come back from them.

I'm a pretty straight talking woman so skip this section if you're happy without any extra stimuli in this department!

The main things to realise, even after all these years, is that it's as rare as 'hens' teeth' for you both 'to arrive at the station at the same time'.

For you 'to arrive at the station' without clitoral stimulation.

For either to 'arrive' if one person is in pain, therefore, investing in a good lube is a *must* for both of you.

For you 'to arrive at the station', (if you haven't so far), with your partner, or in your 'own alone time'. I know this sounds outrageous, but I still speak to women who I know for a fact, have been having sex for years, who have never, or rarely orgasmed. Now, at 46, I'm thinking "why the hell are you still doing it that way, if you don't benefit?!", but hey.

If you're still shy with your partner, then again, I suggest you write them a letter (I will return to this).

I'm very cross with the way that sex education is delivered in general, but back in the day it was worse… it was all 'he puts that there, then semen goes there, then she gets pregnant'!

Terrifying! So you see, our sex education in our generation was by reading Jilly Cooper books etc., but now it's by 50 Shades of what not!

I've spent many years since the publication of that (in my role as a secondary school teacher), explaining to youngsters (15+), that if their boyfriend is expecting all of *that*... then don't and ditch. A girl or woman should never have sex where she's not getting reciprocal attention! However, in the case of this book and chapter, we're all big girls now so we can start to change, explore, experiment and have some fun.

So, back to the letter... if passion has dissipated and the sparkle dulled a little, write this down, acknowledge it and tell him it's not necessarily him (but if it is, don't write the letter, but assess whether it's time to call it a day!).

Tell him how you feel. Explain to him that you need patience, but that you're working on this. Tell him that you may well be ready to "play", but that he is going to *have* to be patient, because, at the moment, you can only "play" when you've set up the game.

Setting up the game...

Your partner needs to know that the 'playground' has to be set up by you, for you, when you want, and that the game may take longer than before.

You and your partner may need to change the schedule of the game, because you're too tired at night, because your IBS is playing up, because you need prep time. Therefore, he must be flexible – but hey, they love it!

Use code words during the day like "I'm off for a read, I'll see you in 5, 10, 15 mins"

They really love this…

a) because it's exciting

b) because they're usually 'up for it'

c) they find your power very sexy

Literally go for a read! My friends introduced me a couple of years ago to the world of 'Erotic Short Stories for Women' by women.

One friend told me about, and shared, her copy of "fairy tales" about erotic fantasies, these are both hilarious and stimulating. This is because a woman's libido is stimulated by her brain and imagination, far more than her bits randomly reminding her!

Fantasies, and in our own head role play, are brilliant and nothing gets things tingling down there than our very own imaginations (given a bit of a head start!).

Obviously now it's easier than ever to download such literary classics, but also and probably very important to you, is to have them on a device in a private library. Nobody really knows what people are reading on electronic devices. You could be reading War and Peace, but it's generally more fun to read a very cheeky, quick version of Alice in Wonderland-ish – very rude but very good/funny.

So we have our imaginations switched on and you can feel stirrings, but blimey, it's still like the Sahara down there. Don't give up, it's just biology letting you down. Now invest in your new BFF (after your Kindle), I introduce you to my friend LUBE…

Now you don't have to physically go into a sex shop or even Anne Summers for this, it's everywhere. Your chemists, Superdrug,

Boots, your supermarket even... BUT...I recommend you combine it with other purchases so 'steady Neddy', let's go nice and anonymously and... ever so delivered in a plain brown box on-line... even Amazon Prime!

This is a very personal choice, but after much discussion with a friend, we go for a silicone based lube – water based like KY and Durex ones are fine, but I prefer the longer lasting, silky smooth, non-sticky silicone versions. I really like a minty one too, because if I'm being self-conscious, because I'm not naturally cleansing as well down there anymore, I just feel more confident and fresh with it. Plus, it really tingles, in a good way!

Hmmm – ok, while we're browsing, we may as well get a decent sized order together. Well-known companies on-line do all sorts, but you can also find good toys on things like Chemistdirect.com

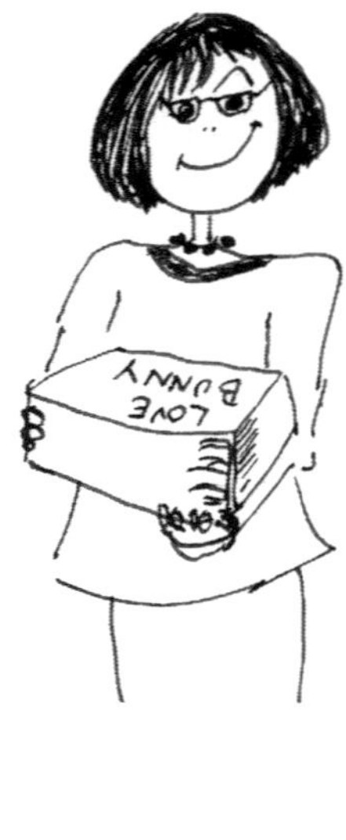

The world is your oyster from here on in. As the short stories will interest you in ideas you never had before, or things you'd like to buzz in or around places you haven't tried before. You practise first – know how you want the game setting out – and then invite your other half to play! Again, the new rules of the game can be in a *love* letter.

I'm not saying that the books or the lube or the 'doodads' or 'gizmo's' work every time. There are some times when I say the immortal words "I'm going for a read..." fully ready with good intentions, and then my body still doesn't respond and I think 'ok, even taking an angle grinder to it isn't going to work today'. That's when I say "oh, can you finish the chapter off" or "match point" – he finishes and we laugh!

Laugh that we can still try.

Laugh that it doesn't matter that the game didn't quite finish the way wanted.

Laugh because we love each other and we literally gave it our best shot.

Laugh and love each other for trying so hard (golly, they're grateful for the effort).

Love each other and send him down to make a nice cup of tea!

I mean, really, it's a very funny pursuit, you can't take it too seriously.

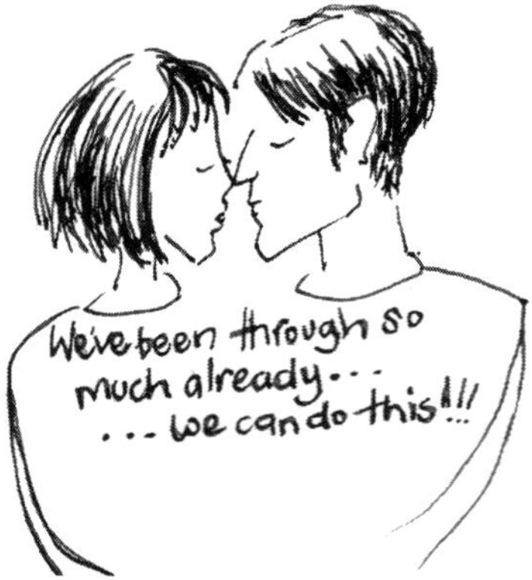
We've been through so
much already...
...we can do this!!!

22
No... You're Not Going MAD!

We all tackle the menopause differently, but what works for me and seems to get good results, is that the more positive I am about it and finding natural solutions, the more I don't feel or even think of myself as menopausal.

Think of it as a symptoms tool box, there will be something that you can try for all of them.

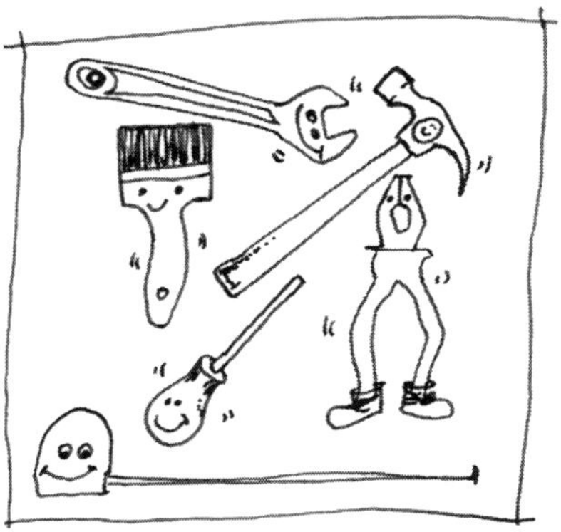

As soon as my hair started to fall out I found 2 x Sea Kelp tablets a day worked (and I still take them). My hair is now even thicker and better than before! It takes a good 8 weeks to start seeing the difference, but persevere because it's worth it.

When my muscles and joints began to ache so much that I couldn't pick up heavy bags, even carrying my handbag hurt (another symptom of the menopause), I found taking 1 x Glucosamine Sulphate a day, all my aches and pains went!

Quite a few months ago I kept waking up feeling anxious, with a feeling of doom or dread that I'd never had before. My husband told me to go to the doctor, but I didn't feel 'ill', I just didn't feel 'right and it was totally out of character.

Then I found out that anxiety is one of the symptoms of menopause, so I take 1 x 150mg Magnesium Citrate in the morning and one at night and all the anxiousness went. Remember 375mg a day is about the maximum your body needs daily but taking a lower dose, twice a day, keeps it in your system.

This is because Magnesium is normally found naturally, as the 4th most abundant hormone in our body, and is known as the 'happy hormone' until the menopause comes along and starts upsetting things. It's needed because it's a calming and relaxing mineral, regulates the nervous system and may help you cope with stress so as to prevent anxiety, fear, nervousness, restlessness and irritability.

Hence, getting it back into your body, can make all the difference in the world to a lot of your symptoms. Citrate is the one that's more easily absorbed by your body. You can also get Magnesium bath flakes (Epsom Salts) and they work well too, on top of a relaxing bath so they are well worth a try.

Get as good a quality as possible with either of these methods, as the cheaper ones can use a lot of 'bulking agents' and this is not good for you at all.

Magnesium is also very protective of your heart and arteries, which is important for anyone experiencing regular anxiety. It's worth a try but you MUST consult your Doctor before taking this, especially if you're on any medication and it's not one to 'up the dose' on thinking that the more you take the better your 'symptoms' might be. It'll just cause you to get diarrhoea! So remember, 375mg a day maximum.

But more on Magnesium later.

We don't always get all the solutions we want to our symptoms. I'm still searching for one that will deal effectively with hot flushes and night sweats for me. I've tried things like Star Flower Oil, Sage and a few others, so I'm now trying magnets to see if that does the trick.

The point to this is that there are a lot of natural remedies that work for a lot of women, and because we're all different it's trial and error with some of your symptoms, as to what will work. But don't give up, you just need to find the one that works for you.

But to be fair, I know that not having a drink every evening and cutting out tea and coffee etc., is all meant to help and even, in some cases, get rid of things like hot flushes, but there are just some things that I enjoy and don't want to cut entirely out of my life.

Cut down, certainly, and this is something we should all consider because, as we get older, our heart, kidneys and liver are getting older too, and the colour of your urine is your body's way of telling you that things are ok, or not!

Very light coloured = OK.

Dark in colour = NOT.

This is your easy daily gauge as to whether you're drinking enough water or not and if you've read chapter 15 hopefully you've already decided to considerably 'up' your intake of water.

I made the decision to try and cut down and only have wine at the weekend. It only took a week or two, not only to get used to it, but to honestly start feeling the benefit of it, which I did. To be honest, I hadn't realised how the units of wine, or cups of tea and coffee had been creeping up over the years!

Not only do I sleep a lot better, but another side effect that I wasn't expecting was that my teeth are a lot whiter now AND my urine is a lot, lot paler! Sorry about that, but I thought important for you to know that, due to what I said in the last paragraph, and after all, it is only you and me here.

I've substituted tea and coffee for water, cold and also hot (which I love) and wine now is usually a white wine spritzer with ice cold sparking water. So you have to way up the 'pro's' and the 'con's' and decide for yourself what your priorities are and what makes you happy.

Another thing... Try and surround yourself with 'kindred spirits' that understand what you're going through.

Have a few around for coffee (or hot water!) and a chat (a moan and a laugh really), it'll make you all feel so much better and stronger to help each other through it, because you all 'get it'. No-one that isn't going through it really does, unless that is, they've watched a family member or friend suffer with the menopause and then they know exactly what you're talking about.

Here's something that sums up the menopause for a lot of us and was written by Nancy Reed and had a load of us agreeing with some of the things she wrote and laughing about it.

She kindly said I could share it with you…

"Menopause definitely has changed a few things for me. Here's a small list.

I once had a beauty mark, now it's a mole with hair growing out of it.

I once had clear skin, now I have acne and am growing a goatee – both at the same time.

I once had pert breasts, now I have two belly warmers.

I once had a thigh gap, now I create so much friction I'm terrified I'll blow up if I have gas.

I once had absolutely no problem getting dressed, made up and ready to go out in one hour. Now I'm lucky if I can put my bra on without getting into an argument with it.

While I've kept a nice head of hair, it seems my ears have become a toupee farmers dream.

I once enjoyed romance, lovemaking and beautiful lingerie. Now a hot cup of tea, a good book, leggings and a baggy sweater make me moan with delight.

I once was a polite and pleasant woman. Now I'm a cross between the girlfriend in Fatal Attraction and the wife in The Postman Always Rings Twice.

I once was a woman who never spoke foul language. Now I'm a woman who can curse a blue streak because the butter wasn't put back, in its proper place, in the refrigerator.

Diahaan Carrol once said that "after forty-five it's all about maintaining oneself" now I know why."

You see? We all go through it, but you know what? Laughter is seriously the best medicine and a huge relief.

What I've found in my personal journey through all of this, my research, putting The Menopause Help Programme together and also this book, is how incredibly awesome a lot of women are…

How you're so supportive.

How you understand, you just "get it".

How a lot of you don't judge.

How you just want to help and be a shoulder to 'moan' on.

You are truly AMAZING.

If it helps you, I've found dozens and dozens and dozens of menopausal symptoms in the research that I've done. I had no idea how varied they are and then, how many times certain ones crop up over and over again (I'll list a few of them below). And how many of us can suffer from any one or more of them.

What I *did* realise, through listening to what was being said, was that the more negative the woman was, the more symptoms she seemed to suffer with, and the more positive the woman was, the fewer symptoms she had!

But whatever they were suffering was REAL to them.

It became quite glaringly obvious too, that an incredible number of women didn't know that a lot of what they were 'feeling' were Menopausal symptoms, until some others said that they were suffering the same things too.

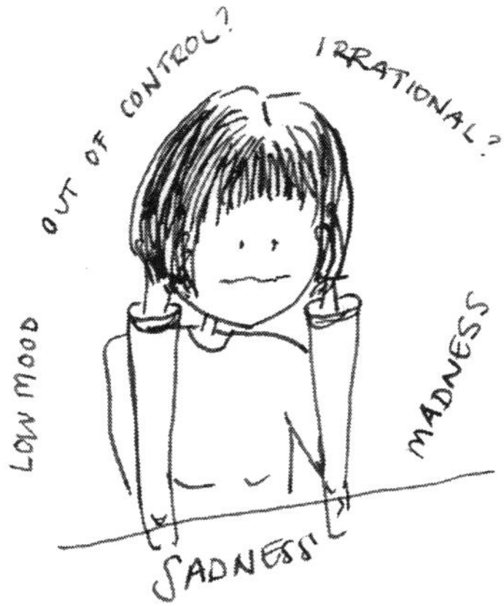

The biggest eye-opener was the relief they felt when they discovered other women out there were feeling a lot of the same symptoms, just like them, and more than that, they were all understanding.

Because of this, I've created a closed support group on Facebook (details at the back of the book) so us women can get the positive help and support that'll get us through this stage and then beyond, as pain free as possible. Because we just need to talk to and support each other. Finding solutions wherever we can and just getting on with life and enjoy it as much as possible. But much more than that, having a giggle.

NOTE: List the remedies that you've tried and what did and didn't work for you...

23 Menopause – Some of What to Expect…

There's sheer relief for women, when they find out that they're not "going mad" when other women totally understand what they're going through.

During my research, I found loads of them that had been to their Doctor, time and again, with no joy. Because, from what I can gather…

* This subject is an absolute mine field.
* There are so many more symptoms than Doctors realise.
* Not all women are the same, and suffer the same.
* It effects women at different ages – there are no rules!
* The longer that women go undiagnosed, the worse they suffer with the menopause (because it seems to start a downward, anxious spiral)
* That women feel like they're "knocking her head against a brick wall", because no-one's 'listening', then who on earth can help her?
* Where does she go, to be understood? For someone to understand that it's not "all in her mind"?
* That what she's going through is VERY REAL, more than a lot of Doctors' realise.
* It's not just a "woman thing". It's *so*, much more than that.

* That it can then affect a woman mentally, as well as physically, the longer it goes on without help.
* That the earlier they are diagnosed or believed to be peri-menopausal the easier it is for them to cope with the years ahead.
* That finding solutions to their symptoms helps give them their life back.
* That the more it's brought out in the open the better it is, not only for the poor women suffering it, but their families. It has a huge knock-on effect when people, and she understands it.
* That for a lot of women, if not most of them, being put on anti-depressants wasn't the answer!

So here, as promised are some menopausal symptoms. But remember, these are only some of them so please don't think you're 'going mad' if you're suffering others that are different and not on this list.

The research I've done has ended up producing an A-Z of Symptoms and Solutions, but anyway, for you now, here are the 25 more 'common' ones...

1) Changing/Irregular Periods - length of cycle, duration of period, lighter/heavier (you might still be able to become pregnant even if you haven't had a period for 1 year!)
2) Hot Flushes/Flashes/Night Sweats (the most common symptom)
3) Weight Gain
4) Lack of Sleep/Insomnia/Lack of Dream Recall

5) Vaginal Dryness
6) Decreased Libido/Sex Drive
7) Mood Swings/Anxiety/Irritability/Depression/Despair
8) Fatigue/Lethargy/Clumsiness
9) Breast Tenderness
10) Bloating/Belching
11) Increased PMS
12) Joint Pains and/or Muscle Pains/Cramps
13) Urgency for the Toilet or Leakage
14) Loss of Confidence
15) Headaches
16) Blood Sugar Crashes - urgency to eat - especially at night!
17) The increased need for Salty, Sugary, Sour or Strong tasting foods
18) Memory Loss/Lack of Concentration
19) Cold Flushes
20) Thinning Hair/Hair Loss
21) Weakened Fingernails
22) Dry Skin/Dry Eyes
23) Change in Body Odour
24) Itchy/Crawly Skin
25) Facial Hair

So as you can see. Knowing that these are some of the symptoms will hopefully help calm you down if you're anxious about anything you're feeling. Please don't expect to experience all of these, you won't. Some will get half a dozen or less, some a bit more.

But what I do know about us, is that when women know about, and understand something, they're a lot less likely to get phased, anxious or worried because we're so much stronger than men realise and we cope, amazingly well.

Just be comforted by the fact that the majority of all women on the planet will get menopausal symptoms when it's the right time for them. Whether that's naturally, or forced (a bit like mine). It doesn't matter. Mother Nature takes over and tries to sort things out.

To give you an example of how BIG this is, at this year of writing, there are 13 million menopausal women in the UK. That's 1/3 of the female population, and it's growing!

Some of us, who are getting a bit fed up, will look to natural remedies (like I did, because 15 years and still going is a long time!). But on that note, because of what I've found to 'cope' with my symptoms, has meant, for me, that I'm not suffering at all with the menopause and the remedies that I take, have allowed me to somewhat "breeze" through this stage of my life a lot more easily than a lot of women and that was the driving force behind Menopause Help and writing this book.

Now before you roll your eyes and say "lucky c**", knowing that it "won't work for me" - WHY NOT? Why won't it work for you? Is there anything that makes you different? You're a woman, who's starting or going through the menopause like the rest of us.

It's a perfectly natural thing (however horrible is it, just like puberty was), but

there's loads of help out there,

there's loads of solutions out there and

there's loads of things you can do to come through this stage as pain free as possible.

But some of us, who get very severe symptoms and really can't cope, look into HRT and there's lots of women out there who absolutely swear by it and said that taking it has given them their life back.

Now I can't really talk about this subject in much detail, I've never gone on it because I wanted to do it as naturally as possible, so I haven't had this experience, but what I have found out is this...

HRT is designed to replace the female sex hormones that naturally decline over a period of months or years during menopause.

There are loads of different types of HRT so there should be one that suits you.

If you're offered a prescription for Premarin, this is a synthetic form of HRT and is made from the urine of pregnant mares. (*pre*gnant *mare*'s urine is the best way to remember this), so anything that has 'Prem' in it, you know where it's come from.

I would advise you research this, or the other types of HRT that you might be offered beforehand so as you're comfortable taking it.

Stopping HRT is not as easy as starting it, so you must consult your Doctor if this is what you want to do, plus the fact that a lot if not all your symptoms could come back with a vengeance when you come off it. But for a lot of women, just the fact that going on it has taken all their symptoms away in many cases, it good enough for them.

But for women who don't want to, or can't take this type of HRT due to their personal choice or a history of breast cancer in their family, then another option they have is a natural 'HRT' (although it isn't, but saying it makes it easier to grasp), is something called 'Bioidentical Hormones'. This is taken from soybeans or yams and their 'structure' is designed to replicate exactly the hormones produced by your body.

These Bioidentical Hormones come as estrogen patches or gel and Utrogestan progesterone capsules. You should be able to get these either from your Doctor or a Menopause Clinic or a Gynecological Consultant at a hospital.

If you're struggling to find where to go for this, then get in touch with me and I'll put you in touch with an expert on this and where you can get it.

If you're considering taking HRT, then you really should carefully discuss the benefits and risks of treatment with your Doctor to see what is right for you. They will take into account your age, medical history, risk factors and personal preferences, along with most probably wanting to know about how the females in your family coped with, or are coping with the menopause.

My advice to you, is thoroughly research HRT in all its forms before you go, so that during what can be a stressful conversation with your Doctor, you are much better armed with the facts to have an outcome that you're happy with.

But, like with everything, you have the right to decide what you want to take and what you don't.

Another thing that a lot of women who come off synthetic HRT are unaware of, is that, as I've said before, if they suddenly stop taking it, they could re-develop menopausal symptoms, which are sometimes even stronger than they were before.

Because Bioidentical Cream Hormones are normally in much lower doses, as far as I know, there are no side effects or withdrawal symptoms and they are out of your system within 24 hours.

You might get to know pretty much what symptoms are going to happen, what days of the month, even if the timing of your period's inconsistent and what happens prior to it will become a good gauge for when you might get your period.

For example, you might be 3 days earlier than 'expected', but you might know the day before because you might have started feeling a bit dizzy, or have fatigue, or have stomach issues etc. - Do you see where I'm going with this?

What would be a good thing for you to do, before you even consider going to the Doctor, is to keep a diary of 'symptoms' when you start noticing changes. You'll know when, because you know your body better than anyone else and you'll just feel that some things aren't quite right and, because you've now read this book, you'll be more aware of what types of symptoms you might be experiencing.

You could either use a paper diary, or a great tool you could look at is a phone app called *'Womanlog.pro'.*

As I said, there are no rules, there's no right or wrong so we can't judge each other.

You know your body better than anyone else, so *you* have to do what's right for *you*.

That also comes true when you keep going to the Doctors because you know 'something isn't right', but the more 'material' or information you have, the easier it should be for you to be diagnosed as menopausal, more quickly, or get rid of your symptoms, as and when they start, naturally.

The Doctor might get you to have a few blood tests, that's because your hormones fluctuate so dramatically over a period of months, so it could be quite a long time before your blood test comes through that you *are* menopausal.

You might want to read and be aware of this...

Something that I've heard from a lot of women who, at the beginning of feeling different symptoms, went to their Doctors about them.

They said they were initially treated for depression and anxiety and prescribed or offered anti-depressants because some Doctors refused to even consider it could be peri-menopause and with a lot of them they were told they couldn't be, because they were too young!

As I said, you know your body and you, better than anyone. If you're not comfortable with this sort of diagnosis, and your

Doctor hasn't found anything 'wrong' with you, then there are other options.

You can try natural remedies and the thing that seems to have the biggest results for a lot of these women is eating a healthier diet and exercising.

It certainly helped me in more ways than one and is definitely something you should consider, as you (and your body) are getting older, that a healthy diet is a lot easier for your body to cope with as it's a lot more 'natural'.

Another thing you might not realise (I certainly didn't – until I started suffering with anxiety!) is how much our body needs Magnesium and how powerful an effect it has on our body, when it decreases! It's thought that there's a link of having lower Magnesium levels to aging and age-related diseases.

Why Magnesium? Because it's a nutrient that the body naturally needs to keep you healthy like your muscles, nerves and making protein and bone (because it balances out calcium and prevents it becoming toxic!).

It also helps keep a steady heart rhythm, a healthy immune system, normal blood sugar levels and blood pressure and is involved in making energy and protein for the body.

It helps with so many other things, including your sleep patterns. It can be found naturally in some foods, including green vegetables, beans and peas, nuts and seeds and whole grains, but unfortunately, over time, food processing practices have essentially stripped Magnesium out of most diets which has caused numerous people to be Magnesium deficient!

It keeps your mood up and keeps you happy, which, I suppose, is why, when we lose Magnesium we can start to feel anxious, and that's what happened to me, until, as I mentioned above, I did, and still do, take 1 x 150mg Magnesium Citrate tablet twice a day and all my anxiety went.

I also back this up with a much healthier diet, including the foods that I've mentioned in chapter 16. But make sure that you don't take any more than about 375mg Magnesium a day (that's why I take a smaller mg dose in capsule form, because I'm topping this up with the foods that I eat) because overdoing it is not good for you and it can give you diarrhoea.

NOTE: List the symptoms you have...

24
Mother Nature Already Has a Lot of the Answers

Here are some natural remedies and solutions that you could try if you're suffering from any of the following...

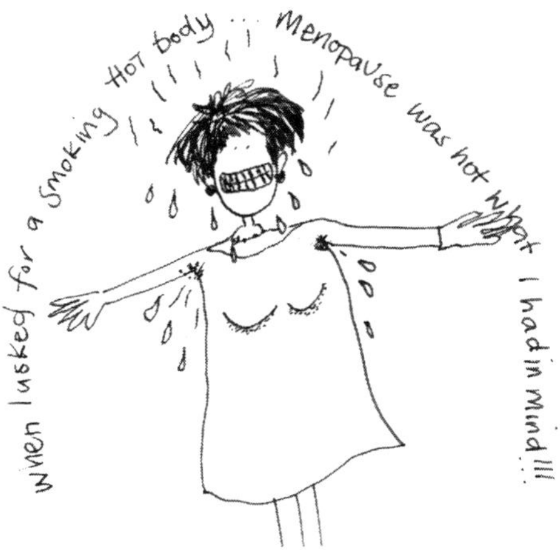
When I asked for a Smoking Hot body... Menopause was not what I had in mind!!!

Irregular Periods	Try eating more fruit and vegetables and less refined sugar and caffeine. Also do all you can to have better sleep and reduce stress in your life (this will help you in so many more areas than your periods).
Hot Flushes	Essential Oil like Clary Sage, Chamomile, Thyme, or Peppermint. For a lot of women, this is a good one if you feel a hot flush coming on and want to nip it in the bud –

put a few drops on a tissue and breath in and rub the Peppermint into your skin on your temples, behind your ears and at the back of your neck.

Some women swear by taking an anti-histamine tablet every day & all their hot flushes went.

Sage capsule daily

Evening Primrose Oil capsule daily

Do the suggestion below with a tiny hot water bottle and put in a zip lock plastic bag in your hand bag for an instant cool down on your chest or the back of your neck.

Night Sweats

Fill a small hot water bottle ½ way with cold water, put it in the freezer and take it to bed with you (wrapped in a hand towel) for an instant cool down.

Sleep in a cool room (preferably with a window open) and with as little on as possible so that its only your skin that has to cool down (this will happen a lot more quickly, than if you have layers on)

Also rub some Peppermint Oil into the soles of your feet when you go to bed.

Aching Joints	1 x Glucosamine Sulphate capsule once a day
Bloating	Avoid Dairy Products, Beans, Apples, Onions, Broccoli, Artificial Sweeteners and Wheat (because we get an intolerance to it as we get older and our body can't digest it).
Anxiety	Magnesium Citrate is the best absorbed and one of the gentlest on the stomach. You can also get Magnesium Flakes (Epsom Salts) for the bath, or a spray that you put on the inside of your elbows and the backs of your knees (be warned that this can stain your bed sheets) as this is the quickest and most direct way to get into your system. *Again, consult your Doctor first if you're on ANY medication.* Lavender Oil Capsules
Thinning Hair	2 x Sea Kelp Tablets once a day
Dry Skin	100% Coconut Oil, Bio Oil, rubbed into your body whilst it's still quite wet from a shower or bath (your skin will absorb more)
Itchy/Crawly Skin	Aqueous Cream

Vaginal Dryness	Over the Counter Creams
Incontinence	Reduce your caffeine intake, balanced diet rich in fruit and vegetables and whole grains, drink at least 6-8 glasses of water a day (delay going to the loo for as long as possible to strengthen your bladder), Pelvic Floor Exercises & wearing a thin pad until your Pelvic Floor strengthens.
Memory Problems	It's important to exercise your brain cells so puzzles, word search, crosswords, anything like that will help. Try putting as many of the foods listed in chapter 10 into your diet as possible. Rosemary Capsules
Dry Eyes	Pharmacies sell a product called 'Hypromellose' which is Artificial Tears (don't use 'eye drops')
Facial Hair	Electrolysis, Facial Hair Product Removal Creams, Strips or an Epilady!
Insomnia	Panax Ginseng has been known to work Avoid caffeine after 2pm as it's a powerful stimulant and takes up to 8 hours for your body to recover from just one cup of coffee! After this time try herbal teas or even hot water.

Weakening Nails	Massage a Vitamin-rich Oil into the base of your nail every night or soak your nails in some Lemon Juice for 5 minutes, dry and then rinse thoroughly and massage in the Vitamin-rich Oil again.
Bags/Wrinkles	Water, water, water. The more the better. Your body needs a minimum of 2-3 litres a day, just to do its job. Any more than that, your body will then use it to break down fat and cellulite! Cup of good quality strong green tea, allow to cool, place in an ice cube tray (half way up) and freeze. When needed, wrap a cube in something soft, gently massage or press under and around your eyes.
Restless/Twitching Legs	Fresh bar or unscented soap, scored on one side with a comb, serrated knife, or your fingernails and place under your bottom sheet (scored side up) by your legs. The ions released should stop your legs twitching. If they start again, re-score the soap.

NOTE: List here what worked for you...

25
NOW is the Time…

Now, this is your call…

For me? I want to be happy, I honestly think that we all have that right.

To look as good as I can, to laugh, make new friends and interests and really enjoy my life as much as possible. I don't want to hurt anyone in the process, but I'm getting older and I want my time, something for me. So what was stopping me trying new or different things, to start getting outside of my comfort zone and doing something just for me?

I wonder if any of this resonates with you too? Was it…

Laziness of taking the first step?

Lack of confidence to try something new?

The worry that people won't like me when they meet me?

Is it really worth the effort (it's so much easier just to stay in).

Can I go out on my own? Am I strong or brave enough?

But if you keep on doing what you're doing, nothing will change! You have to take a deep breath and just take one step in a direction, any direction.

Anything that gets you moving…

You've got to conquer your fears and open the doors to life… and that's exactly what I did. I'll share it with you so that you can see, just how easy it is to start changing your life.

You can make it as easy, comfortable, or challenging as you want. It's your life and your call.

The thing I chose to do first? It was to go to my local WI. Now don't roll your eyes. It was something I could try without any commitment (dip my toe in the water). I was expecting groups of old women knitting 'Dr.Who' style scarfs. How wrong I was...

They were so much younger that I thought they'd be (in the UK, the average age range is from 30 to 70) and there wasn't a knitting needle in sight!

Just chatting, laughter and wonderful women from all walks of life and all there for the same thing – friendship! It took about 3 or 4 visits, before I started to feel more comfortable and less of the 'newbie' as there were new women coming in every month.

It was as easy as that.

It's made a HUGE difference to my life and confidence and given me some of the most amazing friends and I still haven't knitted a scarf! And doing just this one thing, has led me to do other things that I wouldn't have dreamed of doing if I hadn't found out that there are the most wonderful, beautiful, funny people out there that I wouldn't have been lucky enough to meet, if I hadn't taken a chance to find out!

If you try something and it doesn't work? Don't go back – it's easy to pick and choose what does and doesn't suit you. It's your call, so why not try and give it a go? You have no idea how many wonderfully funny people are out there, waiting to meet you.

You had some suggestions in chapter 12 Consider anything that gets you thinking about what you want to do now. As you are now, and what you'd like to become. Once you decide that you want things to change, low and behold, they start changing.

So push the boundaries and enjoy your next chapter...

26
... Time for the 'New You'

Now in this chapter, I talk quite a lot about me, not because I want to, but because the journey I've ended up going on has been so extraordinary that I couldn't find anything to write that might inspire you enough to make a difference to you and your life.

So if it can happen to me – then it can *definitely* happen to you too. Please don't think it can't, because it really can. So read on and try and realise how much your life could change, if you just took some chances...

If you thought you had more time, what would you do?

I saw a sign once that said

"Life isn't about FINDING YOURSELF,

life is about CREATING yourself"

So why not have a list making weekend – how could you change your life for the better?

I'm not going to lie, it takes courage to change, so dig deep and take that first step, but you won't regret it. I did it and it changed my life and ended up by you reading this book and that's just one of the changes that's happened!

So if I can do it for me, you can do it for you too. Remember...

There are no rules, nothing is too big or too small. We're all different and unique and we all have something special to say, tell, show. Whatever it is that's unique to you, and there will be something, you just have to find it. It's out there, waiting for you to take a deep breath and follow your intuition.

Even if it's only one thing, it's the start that's the most important. Remember 'Never Give Up' because anyone can change, either by small steps or a giant leap and you're a lot stronger than you think!

This is your ONE life. Days and then weeks slip by and then you look back at another menopausal year gone and think "how on earth did that happen?".

That was exactly what was happening to me and by changing and trying a few things, my life's changing so much, in more ways than I could have ever imagined, or even felt lucky enough to wish for and I would love that for you too.

So how did my life change? I had no idea but an opportunity came along where my husband, Russ, bought tickets to an Andrew Reynolds (one of the UK's leading entrepreneurs) seminar in the lovely seaside town of Brighton on the south of England coast, and, unbeknown to me, that was where I was going to take the first step and it was literally going to end up re-creating me and my future.

I went along thinking "what the heck, we might learn something". I listened to a load of speakers and one resonated with me, a man called Simon Coulson knew a man called Richard McMunn who is a #1 best-selling author.

Well, the opportunity had just presented itself which lead me taking the biggest leap of faith (giant step) and going for it...

The result? You're reading it!

If I hadn't taken a chance.

If I'd played it safe and never jumped off the cliff of self-doubt, or I'm too old, you wouldn't be reading this.

My life wouldn't have changed beyond anything that I'd ever dreamed of.

The most amazing people would never have come into my life as they have done.

I would never have realised how many incredible, self-giving, wonderful people there are out there and finding out who are the givers, not the takers.

I would never have dreamed that at the age of 58, my life and future would change for ever!

Guess what? We decided to do it again and went to another Andrew Reynolds seminar in Brighton (idiot you might think), but what did I have to lose? You don't need to commit to anything if you don't want to. But someone else cut right through me and off I went again!

His name was Steven Essa, the most amazing and exuberant Australian who talked about creating Webinars. Well, I was hooked.

I was writing a book about telling women how to survive the menopause, thrive, to feel alive and enjoy the next chapter of their life and then the next.

BUT… what if I could SHOW them? How amazing would that be?

The only problem was that I didn't know how to do a Webinar, in fact I didn't even know what one was!

But again, a deep breath and the belief that this had crossed my path for a reason and to be honest, what did I have to lose (ok, the money Russ and I invested), but what if it WORKED, REALLY WORKED?

It's amazing what you're capable of when you've invested in yourself and put 'some skin in the game' as they say, it'll blow you away and totally focus you!

Believe me, it's not all plain sailing. There's been quite a few times of doubt and self-sabotage, "can I really do this", "I'm so out of my comfort zone", but that's where mentors and new friends come into their own and put the wind back under your wings and give you the courage and self-belief to FLY.

Don't expect maybe your family or even some of your friends to understand why you're doing something so out of character. But more importantly, try not to be pressured or influenced into *not* doing something out of character for you that *you* want to do, or resonates with you.

If it feels right for you, (like it did for me) and even if your heart is hammering (like mine was), what have you got to lose by going for it? Until you do this, you'll never know what you're capable of.

Remember you've got ONE life, THIS life…

But the biggest thing to know is that *nobody* was born an expert – but we all know something that could help others and what *you* know or do, can only be told *your* way. There's no one quite like you because *you're* unique, we're all unique in some way. Some are braver to take a leap of faith and do something about it, some aren't.

A friend told me something that really took me by surprise (and might you too) but made absolute sense and that was... "You become the average of the 5 people you spend the most time with". Who are you surrounded by? Something to think about!

Who's putting the wind under your wings to fly?

So my message to you? If you don't TRY, how will you ever KNOW what un-tapped, exciting, wonderful, stupid, funny and life changing opportunities lie within you and in front of you?

If you want to start changing you and your life, I can help you with that if you like with my step-by-step programmes that you can do from home (see the end of this book for the link).

But don't (like me), think that if you're a certain age then it's all just about over and that it's too late...

That no-one will listen to you.

That you'll just be invisible!

HECK NO... NO, NO, NO. This my beautiful friend, is only just the beginning because THERE ARE NO RULES ⍰

Kick the menopause and the 'growing old' into a cocked hat and just GO FOR IT, because your future self will love you for it.

NOTE: List here what you could do that might change your life…

27
Time and Fear!

A friend said to me when I was feeling particularly low and sorry for myself, something that pulled me straight out of my wallowing and I thought, "why the heck not, that's exactly what I'm going to do"...

"F.E.A.R."

Has two meanings

Forget Everything And Run

OR

Face Everything And Rise

"The choice is yours Shelley, so which one are you going to choose?"

So I ask the same thing of you. Which one are you going to choose?

It was powerful and maybe at the time a bit harsh, but it did the trick and made me realise that it *was* my choice.

That we have the immense power to change anything we want. No matter what our age or circumstances.

When I kept thinking negative things like...

"I'm feeling really fed up"

"I don't feel myself"

"I'm feeling really flat"

"Why do I feel so down?"

I had horrible, dull, boring, miserable days.

And then I realised why when I read a random article on 'Mindfulness'. Now don't roll your eyes (because I did that too) thinking here we go, a load of 'woo-woo' stuff, but when I really looked into it, it was so true and everything made sense.

I honestly had no idea that our minds are THAT powerful.

Because I was telling myself that I was "fed up", "down", "bored" etc., that's exactly what I was inviting my day ahead to be and that's exactly what I got. Another boring, same old, day.

I'd been fine before when the family needed me and I was busy from waking up to going to bed. But the girls have gone and are enjoying their lives as young women.

No, I haven't got 'empty nest syndrome' as a lot of other poor women have. I knew that they would leave and I'm delighted that they're being entrepreneurial and getting on with what they want to do.

What I hadn't been expecting was 'TIME'.

'Time' gave me time to think. I now had all this free, spare "ooh I can do anything" time ahead of me, but what I was struggling with, was how to fill it and what to do!

Again, we're all different and some of us love to potter in the garden and go for long walks and that's absolutely perfect. But I tried it and for me, it just wasn't enough.

I'd really enjoyed helping my husband with growing the business, being a wife and mother to our three girls and everything that that entailed over the years, but what I hadn't realised (until I was in my 50's) was how much of 'me' had sort of receded into the background.

I have all this 'time' now, so what the heck was I going to do with it? Does that sound like you too?

You know what? I was BORED! Are you BORED too?

Are you the same and know that you're getting older but you don't 'feel' old?

Now I know what they mean when the say that the 50's are now the new 40's. Mentally and often physically, we're getting younger as we get older, I think that makes sense!

I had far too much time ahead of me just to 'give up' to old age being on the horizon and accept that the menopause is the 'final chapter' in a woman's life.

AS HECK IT IS… OH NO, NOT FOR THIS ONE and you might, along with thousands of other women, feel the same way too.

I know for a lot of women they feel that the menopause is like the Grim Reaper and that's it.

That they're no longer useful, attractive or even noticed. Well you can change most, if not all of that.

Did you know that the most attractive thing on a woman is a smile, and that's just the start to making a difference.

Who are you drawn to? Someone who's smiling, or someone who looks as miserable as sin?

Try it! Next time you pass, or have eye contact with someone, smile at them and I'll bet you they smile back, because not only are they drawn to you, you've drawn something out of them.

It's incredibly contagious.

So...

If you've had enough of feeling sorry for yourself or down, decide to start making changes because...

it will begin to make a difference,

it will help,

it will become very powerful

and then even life changing....

Now. For some of you, all the chapters you've read above will be more than enough to change your life completely.

You'll love the reflection you see when you look in the mirror with your fabulous new hair style.

Because you've mastered doing your makeup and you look 'so good'.

You've lost a bit of weight and it really suits you.

You're so much fitter and healthier and it shows in your skin and eyes.

You've got some hobbies now that you're having so much fun with.

You've met some amazing new friends that are enriching your life more than you thought possible.

You're enjoying having your wardrobe sorted out and have clothes for any occasion and you know you're 'looking amazing'.

You're getting closer to your partner again, and he's starting to understand and support you.

You're being noticed.

You're fun to be with,

and the icing on the cake – YOU'RE ENJOYING LIFE.

It's so nice NOT to be responsible for so much and have time to do things for yourself.

Learn to say "No" to things you can't or don't want to do (the world won't stop, I promise), because now you can dictate things to your own pace.

But. For some others. There might still be something missing...

And that's what I felt. I knew there were things yet to explore, or do, or learn ahead of me. For goodness sake, I don't feel old and I didn't want to live the rest of my life either, worrying about what other people thought, or regretting that I hadn't done something about it.

But what was 'IT'?

Then I knew.

I love learning. I've done it all my life. Anything new, I want to have a go at and see if I can do it. But it went beyond hobbies and interests. It had to be something more…

There are honestly things and people out there that can and will change your life.

Completely…

There's so much out there that you don't know, and that a lot of it isn't there by chance, at all, because 'things', opportunities and people come into your life for a reason.

Now, you might be a lot like me, in that you're not the most blessed with technology. I wasn't, to put it mildly. Ok I could use a mobile phone, send an email and work the microwave (just!), but until you start trying something new, whatever it is, you have no idea what you ARE capable of. It's just good to take a leap of faith and TRY…

That's how my incredible new journey began and how I'm talking to you know, sharing some of the things I know. I say "some", because you never stop learning and growing and I know there'll be loads more things I can and will share with you in the future.

What I'm trying to say is……

It's never too late.

You're never too old.

There's so much out there to be had and to enjoy.

When something crosses your path, maybe, just maybe it's the 'Holy Grail' for you.

WHAT IF ONE OPPORTUNITY COULD CHANGE YOUR ENTIRE LIFE?

That this amazing life isn't a dress rehearsal and we only have one go at it.

And the final thing – *trust in yourself* because you're a lot better, cleverer, smarter and wonderful than maybe you think you are and that right now is *your* time.

28
It's Time to Take Control of Your Life

I can't believe you've read this book to the end and I'm so humbled that you did. It means that you're ready for something amazing and that's brilliant.

It might be a bit scary, but remember 'baby steps' and just like a jigsaw puzzle, it takes time for things to come together, but half the fun is putting those pieces together for the bigger picture.

Now it's your time to have fun, because you know what?

"YOU'RE NEVER TOO OLD TO REINVENT YOURSELF". (Steve Harvey).

Try and make the most of yourself NOW, because it's amazing how easily time just slips by without realising it. We *all* get old, so it's up to you how you want to live the next chapter of your life, how exciting you want it to be and how many years you could be enjoying the 'New You'.

It's never too late to start, because some women are now defying the traditional views of ageing. They want more experiences, more fun, more freedom and they're using their age as an advantage to rebel slightly and do the things they want to do.

Things that make them happy.

But the light at the end of the tunnel (and yes, there is one), is that...

The menopause passes...

It ends...

It stops!

The menopause can put a hard shell around us, but take back control and let that lovely shiny soft centre emerge, just like this drawing – there's something incredibly special and beautiful inside us all.

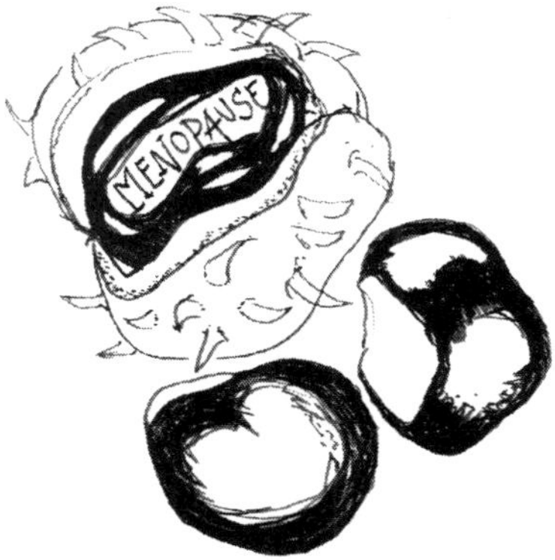

So if you can do as much as possible in your menopausal years to make yourself strong, healthy, attractive and confident, oh boy are you going to have a great life, not only during your menopausal years, but all those ahead of you. If you can use these years the right way, then you're in for the time of your life.

As you get older, you realise that this isn't a dress rehearsal and some of us are just saying "blow it, I'm going to start doing the things that I want to do now" and for a lot of us, and I hope you too, it really works.

Do you know what? There's nothing more flattering than your children's friends saying to them "I wish my Mum was like yours, she's so cool".

Ok, start now, and good luck with wherever it takes you – I wish you all the best and I know that whatever comes your way is exactly what you deserve and could be life changing if you just believe and say “yes”.

Remember, it’s never too late to make a change, but doing something for you is the most important change you can make.

With all good luck my lovely friend, and my very, very best wishes for the ‘New You’.

See you soon

Love

Shelley x

Ps: I would love to know if anything that you’ve done from this has changed your life for the better in any way, however small. Please let me know at ‘shelley@menopausehelp.co.uk.’

If you want to see the Webinar, where I personally go through the Chapters above, please go to…

https://menopausehelp.net/webinar

Something else you might find interesting is “The 3 Things You Must Know About the Menopause” report at…

https://menopausehelp.net/training

Ever thought you’ve got a book in you too? Please go to…

www.best-selling-book.co.uk

ONE MORE THING…

CONGRATULATIONS

You Have Graduated with Flying Colours and are well on your way to the "New You".

Now fill this in and start enjoying becoming the "New You"...

Certificate of Achievement

THIS ACKNOWLEDGES THAT

____

HAS STARTED THE JOURNEY TO THE 'NEW YOU'

Shelley

__________________ __________________

NAME OF AUTHOR

and the most important piece of kit...

Your tool kit of life. There's just about nothing that you can't change or do, so keep looking at this, use your tools lovingly all your life and never stop believing x

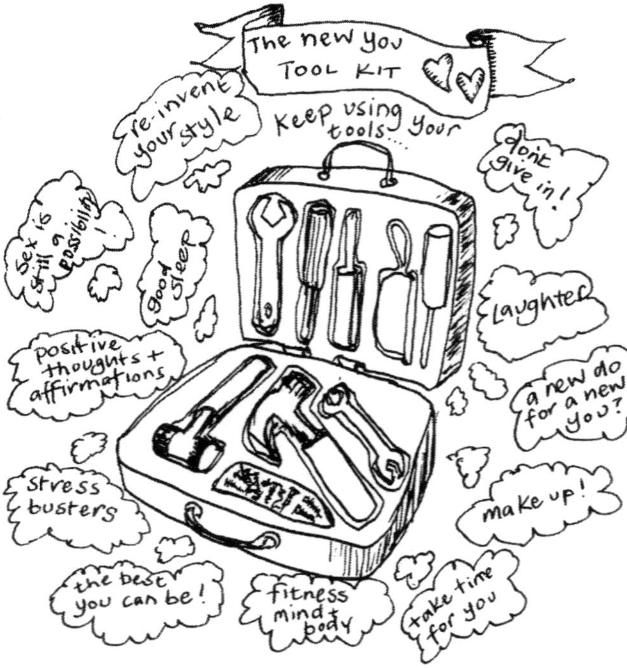

NOTES: For any more notes that you want to make.

27802698R00101

Printed in Great Britain
by Amazon